SAVE +YOUR CHILD'S LIFE!

New Revised Edition

by David Hendin
With an introduction by Peter H. Gott, M.D.

ILLUSTRATED BY JOHN LANE

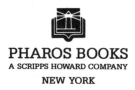

PHAROS BOOKS
A SCRIPPS HOWARD COMPANY

NEW YORK

This edition first published in 1986

Distributed in the United States by
Ballantine Books, a division of Random House, Inc.,
and in Canada by Random House of Canada, Ltd.

Library of Congress Catalog Card Number: 86-61979
Pharos Books ISBN: 0-88687-291-X
Ballantine Books ISBN: 0-345-33718-2

Printed in the United States of America

Pharos Books
A Scripps Howard Company
200 Park Avenue
New York, NY 10166

10 9 8 7 6 5 4 3 2 1

For Sarah, 14, and Benjamin, 11:

I wrote the first edition of this book before you were born,
as part of my research for being your father.

Acknowledgments

The author wishes to thank the following individuals and organizations for the information they have provided which helped in compiling the material necessary to write the book.

American Academy of Pediatrics

American Medical Asociation

American Pharmaceutical Association

Bureau of Product Safety, U.S. Food and Drug Administration

Greater New York Safety Council

Aaron Hendin, M.D.

Jerry Gordon, Division of Research Resources, NIH

Phillip Merwin, New York University Medical School

Metropolitan Life Insurance Company

Michigan Department of Public Health

National Clearinghouse for Poison Control Centers

National Foundation of Sudden Death, Inc.

National Safety Council

Edward Ricciuti

U.S. Coast Guard

U.S. Department of Health, Education and Welfare

Contents

Introduction

We all want to know what to do—not only at the time of an accident, but beforehand as well. David Hendin, a noted medical writer, puts together in this little book all the information that a parent—or prospective parent—needs to know about accidents and poisonings, the number one killer of children. This concise, easy-to-read and fully indexed volume is a must for any adult who raises children, teaches children, or is in contact with children. It should be included in every home and school library.

Save Your Child's Life represents a distillation of the most up-to-date medical knowledge presented in understandable terms with helpful illustrations. Mr. Hendin has organized the chapters for quick reference. Nonetheless, parents will want to familiarize themselves with the methods he describes in order to prevent accidents and know what to do if a crisis occurs.

The purpose of this book is clearly prevention. Danger areas of home and garden are portrayed in a manner that will enable any adult to reduce hazards to children. In our technological society, we are literally surrounded by seemingly innocuous substances that can cause pain, and even death—substances that we would not ordinarily think of as toxic or dangerous. Mr. Hendin outlines a common sense approach to childhood emergencies, and then, as a piece de resistance, he devotes an entire chapter to the babysitter.

Save Your Child's Life is a consumer-oriented book. It tells us about ourselves. More importantly, it tells us about our most cherished possession: our children. Read it. Learn it. Commit its instructions to memory. Use it for reference. The child you save may be your own.

Peter H. Gott, M.D.
Connecticut, 1985

An Important Foreword

A lot has changed since I first wrote this book in 1972. Child-resistant bottle caps, safer toys, better-educated parents, more responsible toy manufacturers, and government regulations have helped to cut dramatically the number of childhood deaths by poisoning or other accidents. Still, thousands of children die every year, and hundreds of thousands more are injured. We can do better.

Even today there are parents who would not know what to do if their child swallowed a poison or stopped breathing. Nobody knows how many children still die when quick, deliberate action might have saved them.

Many parents cannot take the time for a first aid course, or to read a 300-page book on the subject. But you should be able to read this little book in one evening. I suggest you do that—read it through. Then put it in a place where you can get to it quickly.

You will want to follow most, if not all, of the precautions and recommendations for poison-proofing and accident-proofing your home. Do these things right away. One day's wait might be fatal to your child.

In the last dozen years I have received many letters from parents who have followed the advice in this book and who thanked me for it. I even had a letter from one mother who complained that while she was implementing our poison-proofing program, her 2-year-old tried to eat her copy of this book. No harm was done, except to the book, I am happy to report.

When and if an emergency does arise, keep calm. This will be helpful both to you and to the injured child. If no doctor or first aid professional is available, you should have the knowledge to take command of the situation.

1. Keep calm. Right now, you are in charge. You can save a life!

2. Size up the problem.

3. Call the doctor, police, hospital or poison control center.

4. If you must administer first aid, give it quickly and deliberately.

Remember, if an accident occurs and you can't contact your doctor immediately, take your child to the nearest hospital emergency room. Your doctor will probably ask you to meet him there anyway. When getting to a doctor or hospital during an emergency is impossible, then—and only then—should you begin to apply first aid.

I hope you never have to try to save a life. But you will be able to rest easier knowing that you have information you need at your fingertips.

David Hendin
New York, 1985

CHAPTER ONE

The Kiss of Life

When "Dead" Is Really Alive

The AUTHOR...promises to pay the reward of ONE GUINEA to nurses or other attendants, on any child or grown person returning to life by their humane attention, provided the fact is ascertained by a gentleman of the faculty, or attested by three credible persons; and in hopes of exciting a universal attention to a subject of much importance to mankind.

The above offer was made in 1780 in an "Address to the Public" of William Hawes of London's Royal Humane Society. The goal of this and similar organizations was to save the lives of persons who had been drowned, struck by lightning or suffocated and thus thought to be dead. It was with his own money that Hawes was willing to pay those who brought him drowned people within a short time after immersion.

The founders of the "humane" movement learned that they could sometimes restore these "dead" people to life. The victims, of course, weren't really dead at all, but for hundreds of years a person was thought to be dead as soon as his heartbeat and breathing stopped. *We know today that this is not always true.*

As often happens in the case of new discoveries and theories, some scientists of the day laughed at the dedicated men of the humane societies and their crude methods of artificial respiration.

In 1790, Dr. Benjamin Waterhouse told the annual meeting of the Massachusetts Humane Society that "To blow in one's own breath into the lungs of another is an absurd and pernicious practice."

Fortunately for us, all physicians and scientists did not agree with Dr. Waterhouse. Today, the once-controversial "humane" practice is called mouth-to-mouth breathing, or artificial respiration. Commonly taught to physicians and laymen alike, this "kiss of life" has been responsible for saving many thousands of lives, and will save many more.

Today, if William Hawes of London had to pay one guinea, or less than a couple of dollars, to every proven case of a child or adult revived by mouth-to-mouth breathing, he would be a poor man in a short time.

The mouth-to-mouth breathing technique, as well as external cardiac (heart) massage, are easy to learn and should be known by every parent; indeed every person capable of understanding and applying them should be informed.

The reason is, as the humane movement founders helped us learn, that a person who has stopped breathing or whose heart has stopped beating may not be dead. The person may not die for several minutes.

"I remember," Dr. William P. Williamson has written in the *Journal of the American Medical Association,* "when cessation of heartbeat was an observation on which we simply pronounced the patient dead; now, this is a medical syndrome known as cardiac arrest. Cessation of respiration is also a symptom formerly implying death, which can (also) now be corrected..."

Many cases of "deaths" from heart stoppage or respiration cessation occur today—often during surgery—and most hospitals maintain emergency warning systems which are attached to the patient. Around-the-clock duty crews of specialists with resuscitation equipment stand ready to move into action as soon as an alarm signals. One patient died by the old "heart stoppage definition" *for more than 90 times,* but five years later he was carrying on an active life wearing a cardiac pacemaker to assure satisfactory heart function.

A person who has stopped breathing, and whose heart has stopped beating, may not be dead. He or she may become dead if breathing and circulation stop for more than about three minutes, thus starving the brain of the oxygen it needs to operate. The important part is that there are a *precious few minutes* between the time that heart and breathing stop and actual death.

Mouth-to-Mouth

It is during those few minutes that a parent, friend, or pass-er-by can apply a kiss of life more magical and much more important than the kiss Prince Charming gave to Snow White. Interestingly enough, since many fairy tales are based on some sort of fact, it is possible that Snow White had been temporarily paralyzed by a poison, and the Prince was able to maintain her life by mouth-to-mouth breathing.

When a person stops breathing and is suffocated, it is called asphyxiation. This may occur because of choking, electric shock, suffocation, poison gas, drowning or any number of other reasons. Whatever the reason, time is precious. The person will die unless artificial breathing is started rapidly. The delay of only a few seconds may be the difference between life and death.

Aside from a halt in the breathing, other symptoms of asphyxiation are blueness of skin or, in the cases of some poisonings, very shallow breathing.

What to Do

If a child stops breathing, and you are nearby, here is what to do. First and foremost, although it always sounds trite, *keep calm*. You are the only person who knows what to do and how to control the situation; if you panic, you may make mistakes and cause delays.

Start respiration immediately. Do not delay even to phone for help, loosen clothes, remove wet clothes, or move the child to another location. These things can all be done after the child begins breathing again, or by another person. *The most important thing is to get air into the child's lungs.*

Once artificial respiration is begun it should be continued for at least four hours without stopping OR until the patient begins breathing on his own OR until the patient is pronounced dead by a doctor. (If another person is available, you may take 10- or 15-minute shifts giving mouth-to-mouth breathing.)

How to Apply the Kiss of Life

1. Turn the child on his or her back.

2. Quickly remove any foreign matter, such as gum, food, vomitus, or mucus from the mouth. Turn his head to the side and use your fingers to remove all obstructions. (Figure 1.)

3. Put one of your hands under the child's neck and the other under his chin. Pull the chin upward until the head is tilted back as far as possible. This assures keeping the air passages to the lungs open during your revival efforts. (Figure 2.)

4. Place your mouth tightly over the child's mouth and nose. In the case of an older child or adult, put your mouth tightly over the victim's mouth and pinch the nostrils to prevent leakage of air. Otherwise, all of the air you breathe into the mouth may come out the nose. (You may use a handkerchief between your mouth and the victim's, but make sure the seal is tight so air does not escape.) (Figure 3.)

5. Breathe into the child's mouth and nose until you see his or her chest rise. If the air passages are not clear, you may notice that you have blown the child's stomach up with air. This is not dangerous and is easily remedied by applying pressure on the stomach with the palm of one hand. This will expel the air, but may also cause some vomiting, so be ready to turn the child's head to the side again to clean out the mouth with your fingers.

6. Remove your mouth and listen for the sound of returning air. If you don't hear this, recheck the victim's chin and head position. If you still don't get an air exchange, turn the child on his side and slap him on the back between the shoulder blades to dislodge any foreign matter that may be in the throat. Again clean out mouth obstructions. (Figure 4.)

7. Repeat the breathing. Remove your mouth from the

child's mouth and nose each time to allow air to escape. For a small child, take relatively short breaths and repeat *about 20 times per minute.* For an adult, breathe vigorously *about 12 times each minute.*

8. Continue mouth-to-mouth until:

- The child begins breathing on her own, OR
- For at least four hours, OR
- Until the patient is pronounced dead by a doctor.

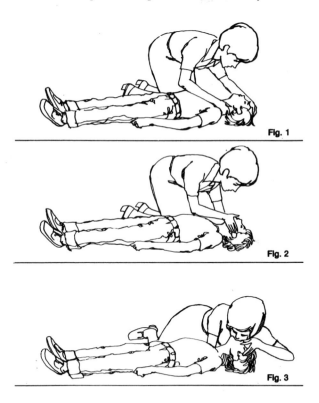

Fig. 1

Fig. 2

Fig. 3

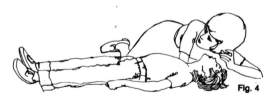

Fig. 4

If the child does begin to breathe on his or her own again, you may congratulate yourself. But DO NOT become over-confident. Be prepared to restart breathing aid if it is needed.

Heart Massage

After the first five or six breaths in mouth-to-mouth breathing have been administered, you should check to see if external cardiac massage should be started.

This is necessary ONLY if the heart has stopped beating. In many cases the mouth-to-mouth breathing itself will be enough to start the heart beating again.

To see if the heart is beating check for a pulse. The most easily accessible pulse for this is the carotid in the neck. This is a large artery in the neck that runs on either side of the Adam's apple. You may practice by finding and feeling your own. If there is no pulse, begin external cardiac massage.

1. Place the heel of your hand on the lower part of the breast bone (Figure 5) and the other hand on top of the first. Since a young child's chest is not as strong as an adult's, external heart massage in infants can be done with two fingers. In older children up to age 10, one hand is usually enough. (Figure 6.)

2. With the weight of your upper body, push down on the heel of your hand (or on your fingers in the case of a baby). The breast bone should move downward an inch or an inch and a half, depending on the age of the patient. (Figure 7).

3. Release pressure quickly. Repeat 80 to 100 times per minute in children and 60 to 80 times per minute in adults.

4. Keep your fingers away from the ribs to avoid fractures.

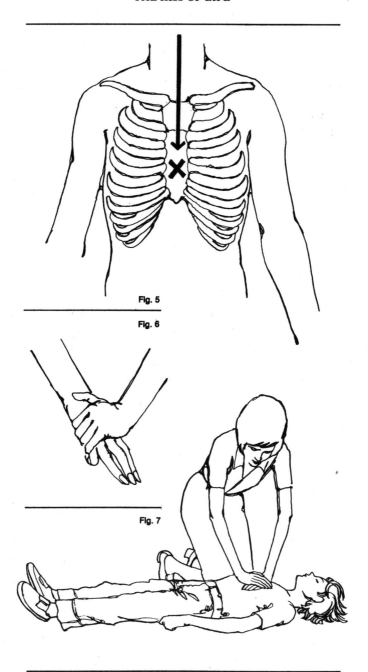

Fig. 5

Fig. 6

Fig. 7

Now you may ask a good, and very important, question: If my child has stopped breathing and his heart has stopped beating, how can I do all of these things at the same time?

The answer is you can, IF you are already familiar with the emergency procedure. IF A CHILD HAS STOPPED BREATHING, DO NOT TAKE TIME TO CALL FOR HELP. BEGIN RESUSCITATION IMMEDIATELY. If another person is available, send him or her for help.

If you are the only person present and you must administer both mouth-to-mouth breathing and external heart massage, here is the procedure:

First give five or six lung inflations, then switch to external heart massage. Interrupt the external massage every 20 to 30 beats to give five or six lung inflations.

If there is a second person present, he or she can administer external cardiac massage while you give the "kiss of life."

If there is a third person present, he can monitor the child's pulse to check the adequacy of your procedure.

Keep calm. You now know and understand the procedures of external heart massage and mouth-to-mouth breathing. You can save a life. In an emergency, if no physician or expert is present, take control of the situation. Your calm and deliberate actions will be of great comfort to others. You will help others get control of themselves: they will then be in a position to follow your instructions.

CHAPTER TWO

Poisons in Your Home

Borgia's Delight

The infamous Borgia family—known for their plots and poison murders in 15th-century Italy—would undoubtedly be delighted with the number of poisons found in the average North American home today.

There are more than half a million different kinds of dangerous medicines, cleaning aids, cosmetic aids, pesticides, and other household products and substances that have been swallowed by children. Your home contains hundreds of them. Many of these substances are not even recognized as dangerous by many adults.

This year alone some 250,000 children will swallow poisonous materials. Half of them will be seriously injured, and at least 200 children will die from poisoning. Will your child be one of them?

Don't Take a Chance

When the television weatherman reports that there is a 90 percent chance of rain on a given day, you will carry an umbrella to work to protect yourself from getting wet.

But when you are told that there is a 100 percent chance that your toddler will explore your house *every day*, what will you do? You will, of course, say that you will watch your child every minute. But that is impossible. *Fully 95 percent* of the reported cases of accidental poisonings have occurred when the children were supposedly under the supervision of parents or other adults. Moreover, 90 percent of all reported cases of poisoning involve children 5 years old and younger.

You *must* poison-proof your home—and do it today. Don't postpone this simple, vital task. If you do, your child may suffer. For further insurance you must learn some basic first aid measures to treat poisoning. No matter how careful you are, your curious child is bound to find something to put into his mouth. Be prepared.

Remember, young children will eat and drink almost anything. Youngsters have been known to drink full containers of kerosene and not be bothered at all by the taste. When a child finds something new, it often goes right into his or her mouth. When your child does this, it does not mean that you have a bad child; this is the child's way of learning about things. You must teach your child as early as possible not to put things into his or her mouth and not to eat or drink things that you have not given the child specifically as food or medicine.

Medicine Isn't Candy

Medicine is not candy. Never call it that to entice a child to take it. Remember that cough syrups can look like soft drinks and many coated medicine tablets can look like candy-coated chocolates or other sweets. Children's aspirin and aspirin substitutes have a pleasant candy flavor so children will take them more readily. Make it clear to youngsters that this is medicine, not candy, and explain what medicine is and when it should be taken (only when a parent gives it).

Child-resistant caps on bottles, mandated by Congress in 1970 for substances that pose a threat to children, have had a dramatic impact on the number of childhood poisonings. Total deaths to children under 5 have decreased an overwhelming 75 percent since the law was passed requiring them, and aspirin related deaths in children have declined 87 percent. These closures may be a minor inconvenience for you, but they may very well *Save Your Child's Life!*

The Poisonous Grandparents

Thirty-six percent of all prescription drugs swallowed by children under age 5 involve a grandparent's medication, according to the U.S. Consumer Product Safety Commission.

This surprising statistic is probably due to the fact that grandparents often request bottles with regular tops instead of the child-resistant variety. Grandparents often justify this because they don't have children living with them anymore and, therefore, would like to avoid this inconvenience.

However, many children under age 5 often gain access to their grandparents' medication when visiting them or when grandparents visit their grandchildren. Even though it is inconvenient, grandparents should use child-resistant bottle-top closures whenever children are, or may be, around.

Prevention, the Only Sure Cure

Here are some more suggestions for poison-proofing your home:

✔ **Keep all products in their original containers.** If you put antifreeze, paints or pesticides into soft drink bottles, milk bottles, cans or cups, your child may mistake these deadly poisons for the good and healthful products that normally come in these containers.

✔ **Destroy all old products.** Pour the contents of containers down the drain or toilet and rinse the container before you throw it away. Never put a full container into the trash can.

✔ **Read the labels of all products you use around the home.** These labels have been written for your safety and protection. *Remember* that your young child cannot read, so keep all dangerous products out of reach.

✔ **Keep food and household products in separate places.** Cleaning fluids, lye soaps, and insecticides may be confused with food or medicine. Don't let your child die because of a case of mistaken identity.

✔ **Make sure your medicine cabinets are locked or well out of reach.** And remember, children are climbers.

✔ **Make sure all cleaners, paints, and other chemicals are stored away just as carefully as medicines.**

✔ **Whenever you take a bottle of aspirin or other medicine out to use, always return that bottle to safe storage immediately.** Don't leave these killers around even for a "few minutes," because it only takes a few seconds for a child to find and swallow them.

✔ **Buy medicine with child-proof tops for double protection, but DO NOT be overly confident in these protection devices.** Safety lock tops are made so they require two or more separate motions to remove them from the bottle. But your child may figure this out. Furthermore, what he cannot open with his mouth he may throw down and break or get into some other way.

✔ **Make sure you cleaned out or locked all under-the-sink cabinets in the bathroom and kitchen.** Clean out or lock all accessible shelves in other storage areas.

✔ **Never leave medicines (aspirin, tranquilizers, birth control pills) lying around on bedside tables, or on other table tops, or in low drawers.**

✔ **Be careful where you leave your purse if you have medicine in it.**

✔ **Be especially careful with medicines and other poisonous chemicals when you move or go on vacations.** These are times when a child can easily catch you off-guard because of the bustle of activity.

✔ **Turn on the light, and make sure you are awake, whenever giving or taking medicine.**

✔ **Remember that when you go visiting ALL OF THE SAME RULES APPLY.** Keep your child in sight, especially in the homes of older persons where pills and other medications are more likely to be left out in the open.

✔ **Remember that as far as poisoning and safety in the home are concerned, there is no doubt that:** PREVENTION IS THE ONLY SURE CURE.

Know Those Poisons

Aspirin is by far the most common poisoner of young children, responsible for many thousands of poisonings every year.

The next 10 most common poisons that affect children are:

Other medicines

Soaps, detergents and cleaners

Disinfectants and deodorizers

Insecticides

Bleach

Glues and adhesives

Acids and alkalies (lye)

Liquid floor and furniture polish and wax

Cosmetic lotions and creams

Signs of Poisoning

If you think your child has swallowed any poisonous substance, immediately call your nearest poison control center (listed on pages 18 to 25) for advice. In this type of an emergency, a call to your doctor or hospital would be second choice, because the poison control center personnel have experience and access to information that most physicians and even hospitals would not have immediately at hand.

Here are some important signs of poisoning. Watch for them in your children:

Overstimulation

Drowsiness

Shallow breathing

Unconsciousness

Nausea

Convulsions

Stomach cramps

Heavy perspiration

Burns on hands and mouth

Dizziness

Changes in skin color

Also watch for:

Unusual stains on skin or clothes

Sudden changes in a child's behavior

Open bottles of chemicals or medicines out of place.

Don't be surprised if your child wakes you up early one morning, or comes to you in the middle of the day, and says, "Baby eat candy." One 2-year-old woke his father with those three words. The child had devoured an entire bottle of thyroid tablets, which he found while exploring the "out of reach" kitchen cabinets. Luckily the child got quick first aid and was not seriously harmed.

If your child gives you any indication that he or she has eaten anything that may be poisonous, act quickly. Speed is the most important factor in first aid for poisoning.

What to Do for Poisoning

Here are a few words that, according to the American Association of Poison Control Centers (AAPCC), will help you save your child's life in case of poisoning:

> In ALL cases it is important to remember to get the poison out OR to dilute the poison. REMEMBER—if anyone swallows poison it is an emergency. (Any nonfood substance is a potential poison.) Always call for help promptly.

If you suspect that a child has eaten a poisonous substance, the AAPCC says you must:

1. Call the Poison Control Center, doctor, or hospital immediately. Give them all the information you have about the poison and the child. Write down and follow their directions.

2. If you cannot reach any of the above, don't waste any more time trying. If another person is available, let him do the calling while you DILUTE THE POISON. Do this by giving the child a glass or two of milk or water. It is important to dilute the poison before you induce vomiting.

3. Make the child vomit if you have been directed to do so by the Poison Control Center, doctor, or hospital. But do not induce vomiting if:

- The child is unconscious or having fits
- The swallowed poison is a strong corrosive (such as ammonia, bleach, lye products, sulfuric, nitric, or hydrochloric acids)
- The swallowed poison contains kerosene, gasoline or other petroleum products (unless it also contained a dangerous insecticide which must be removed). Some common petroleum products include benzene, liquid furniture, and metal polish, turpentine and oven cleaners

Do not make the child vomit if he has eaten any of the above. Instead, if he is conscious, give him a glass of milk (fresh or canned) and get him to the nearest hospital. Vomiting should not be induced in these cases because the strong chemicals may cause more harm when they are regurgitated. Lye may cause the food pipe to rupture and petroleum products may damage the child's lungs.

*   *   *

If the situation calls for you to make the child vomit:

1. Give one tablespoon of Syrup of Ipecac (be sure you ask your druggist for *Syrup* of Ipecac) to a child older than one year. Also give the child at least one cup of water. If no vomiting occurs after 20 minutes, this procedure may be repeated, but repeat it only once unless otherwise directed by a doctor.

2. If you do not have Syrup of Ipecac, you can try to make the child vomit by tickling the back of his throat with a finger or spoon after having him drink lukewarm water.

3. Do not waste time waiting for the child to vomit if he does not do so right away. Take him immediately to a doctor or hospital emergency room. Bring the container or package from which the poison came, and leave any remaining sample of the poison intact.

4. After the child has vomited, you may give him a glass of milk or water to help dilute any remaining poison and protect his stomach.

*   *   *

When taking your child to the hospital, keep the child warm and comfortable. Keep airways open and be sure the child does not choke on the vomitus.

Keep yourself calm. If you are excited, your child may also panic and be more seriously harmed.

In all suspected cases of poisoning, keep watching for signs of shock (see page 53). If shock does occur, TREAT THE POISONING FIRST, and then the symptoms of shock.

If the child's breathing has stopped, apply mouth-to-mouth breathing as described on page 4.

Watch Out for Inhalation Poisoning

Poisonous gases are not as uncommon around the home as you might think. Beware of pesticide and other noxious sprays, as well as benzene and carbon tetrachloride fumes. Be sure to turn off gas burners and stoves after use. Never use charcoal barbecue grills inside the house or in any unventilated area. Never run a car, motorcycle, lawn mower or any other kind of internal combustion engine in a closed area.

In case your child becomes a victim of inhalation poisoning, you must:

1. Ventilate the area. Do this by opening a door or window. Break a window if necessary. Otherwise, the rescuer may actually become a victim.

2. Move the child away from exposure to the fumes.

3. Loosen clothing.

4. Call the doctor, police, or hospital. Better still, let someone else call while you give all your attention to the child.

5. If the child is not breathing, BEGIN MOUTH-TO-MOUTH BREATHING and external heart massage (if needed) as described on page 6.

6. Keep the child quiet and do not give him food or drink.

7. Watch for signs of shock, and treat if necessary (see page 53).

8. Get the child to a medical facility promptly.

Lead Poisoning Can Be Fatal

Lead poisoning maims and kills children. They get lead poisoning from eating little bits of paint over a period of time. The lead accumulates in the body and when it reaches a certain level begins to cause brain damage. The child may become mentally retarded or die.

When you buy paint for your home, make sure it does not

have a lead base. Many old houses and apartments have layers of lead paint on the ceiling, walls and woodwork. When the paint chips, or bits of plaster fall, there is a real danger that babies or your children will try to eat it. This poison tastes sweet like candy, so a child is likely to keep eating it. Keep your home free of paint and plaster chips, and all lead base paints.

If you have seen your child putting chips of paint or plaster into his mouth, you must take the child to a doctor, clinic or hospital as soon as possible. Your child will then be tested for lead in his body. In the early stages of lead poisoning, the child may not seem to be sick. But don't wait for signs of this kind of poisoning to get rid of lead-based paint and plastered areas.

✔ **Does your child chew on painted window sills or painted railings?**

✔ **Does he or she seem to be especially cranky?**

✔ **Does the child throw up or have frequent stomach aches?**

All of these may be signs of lead poisoning. Take your child to a doctor's office or a clinic.

Poison Control Centers

There are about 380 poison control centers in the United States ready to provide you emergency information for treating poisonings. Many of the centers have toll-free lines. Some of them even have the TTY system for communicating with deaf persons. In the case of a poisoning emergency, you should immediately call the poison control center nearest to you. Physicians or the local hospital are second choice, since they do not have as much information or such experienced personnel readily available.

ALABAMA

BIRMINGHAM
The Children's Hospital of Birmingham
1601 6th Ave., South
Birmingham, AL 35233
205 933-4050
800 292-6678 (Statewide)

TUSCALOOSA
The Alabama Poison Control Center
Druid City Hospital
809 University Blvd, East
Tuscaloosa, AL 34501
205 345-0600
800 462-0800

ALASKA

ANCHORAGE
Anchorage Poison Center
Providence Hospital
3200 Providence Drive
Anchorage, AK 99504
907 274-6535

FAIRBANKS
Fairbanks Poison Center
Fairbanks Memorial Hospital
1650 Cowles
Fairbanks, AK 99701
907 456-7182

ARIZONA

FLAGSTAFF
Flagstaff Hospital and Medical Center of N. Arizona
1215 N. Beaver Street
Flagstaff, AZ 86001
602 779-0555

PHOENIX
St. Luke's Hospital and Medical Center
525 North 18th Street
Phoenix, AZ 85006
602 253-3334

TUCSON
Arizona Poison and Drug Information Center
Arizona Health Sciences Ctr.
University of Arizona
Tucson, AZ 85724
602 626-6016
800 362-0101 (Statewide)

ARKANSAS

FORT SMITH
St. Edward Mercy Medical Ctr.
Emergency Room
7301 Rogers Avenue
Fort Smith, AR 72903
501 452-5100 Ext. 2401

LITTLE ROCK
University of Arkansas Medical Center
Emergency Room
4301 W. Markham Street
Little Rock, AR 72201
501 661-6161

PINE BLUFF
Jefferson Regional Medical Ctr.
Emergency Department
1515 West 42nd Avenue
Pine Bluff, AR 71601
501 541-7111

CALIFORNIA

FRESNO
Central Valley Regional Poison Control Center
Fresno Community Hospital
Fresno & R Streets
Fresno, CA 93715
209 445-1222

LOS ANGELES
Los Angeles County Medical Association Regional Poison Information Center
1925 Wilshire Blvd.
Los Angeles, CA 90057
213 484-5151

OAKLAND
Children's Hospital Medical Center of N. California
51st & Grove Streets
Oakland, CA 94609
415 428-3248

SACRAMENTO
Sacramento Medical Center
Univ. of California at Davis Poison Control Center
2315 Stockton Blvd.
Sacramento, CA 95817
916 453-3692
800 852-7221 (N. CA)

SAN DIEGO
San Diego Regional Poison Center
Univ. of Calif. at San Diego Medical Center
225 W. Dickinson Street
San Diego, CA 92103
619 294-6000

SAN FRANCISCO
San Francisco Bay Area Regional Poison Control Ctr.
Room 1E 86
San Francisco General Hospital
1001 Potrero Avenue
San Francisco, CA 94110
415 666-2845
800 792-0720 (N. CA)

SAN JOSE
Central-Coast Counties Regional Poison Control Ctr.
Santa Clara Valley Medical Ctr.
751 S. Bascom Avenue
San Jose, CA 95128
408 279-5112
800 662-9886 (Statewide)

COLORADO

DENVER
Rocky Mountain Poison Ctr.
Denver General Hospital
W. 8th Avenue & Cherokee Sts.
Denver, CO 80204
303 629-1123
800 332-3073

CONNECTICUT

BRIDGEPORT
Bridgeport Hospital
267 Grant Street
Bridgeport, CT 06602
203 384-3566

St. Vincent's Medical Ctr.
2800 Main Street
Bridgeport, CT 06606
203 576-5178

FARMINGTON
Connecticut Poison Control Center
University of Connecticut Health Center
Farmington, CT 06032
203 674-3456

MIDDLETOWN	Middlesex Memorial Hospital, 28 Crescent Street, Middletown, CT 06457	203 344-6684
NEW HAVEN	The Hospital of St. Raphael, 1450 Chapel Street, New Haven, CT 06511	203 789-3464
	Yale–New Haven Hospital, Department of Pediatrics, Pediatric Emergency Room, 20 York Street, New Haven, CT 06504	203 785-2222
NORWALK	Department of Emergency Medicine, Norwalk Hospital, Maple Street, Norwalk, CT 06856	203 852-2160
DELAWARE		
WILMINGTON	Wilmington Medical Center, Delaware Division, 501 W. 14th Street, Wilmington, DE 19899	302 655-3389
DISTRICT OF COLUMBIA		
WASHINGTON	National Capitol Poison Ctr. Georgetown University Hospital, 3800 Reservoir Road, Washington, DC 20007	202 625-3333
FLORIDA		
DAYTONA BEACH	Halifax Hospital, Emergency Department, P. O. Box 1990, Daytona Beach, FL 32014	904 258-1513
FT. LAUDERDALE	Broward General Medical Ctr. Poison Control Center, 1600 S. Andrews Avenue, Ft. Lauderdale, FL 33316	305 463-3131 Ext. 1955/6
FORT MYERS	Lee Memorial Hospital, 2776 Cleveland Avenue, P. O. Drawer 2218, Fort Myers, FL 33902	813 334-5287
PENSACOLA	Gulf Region Poison Ctr. Baptist Hospital, P. O. Box 17500, Pensacola, FL 32522	904 434-4611, 1-800 874-1555 (Out of State), 1-800 342-3222 (Statewide)
TALLAHASSEE	Tallahassee Memorial Regional Medical Center, 1300 Miccosukee Road, Tallahassee, FL 32304	904 681-5411
TAMPA	Tampa Bay Regional Poison Control Center, Tampa General Hospital, Davis Island, Tampa, FL 33606	813 251-6995, 800 282-3171 (Statewide)
GEORGIA		
ATLANTA	Georgia Poison Control Ctr. Grady Memorial Hospital, Box 26066, 80 Butler Street, S. E., Atlanta, GA 30305	404 588-4400, 800 282-5846 (Statewide), 404 525-3323 (TTY)
COLUMBUS	The Medical Center, 710 Center Street, Columbus, GA 31902	404 571-1080
MACON	Medical Center of Central Georgia, Regional Poison Control Ctr., 777 Hemlock Street, Macon, GA 31201	912 744-1427
SAVANNAH	Savannah Regional EMS Poison Center, Dept. of Emergency Medicine, Memorial Medical Center, P. O. Box 23089, Savannah, GA 31403	912 355-5228
GUAM		
AGANA	Pharmacy Service, Box 7667, U. S. Naval Regional Medical Center (Guam), FPO San Francisco, CA 96630	344-9265 Ext. 9354
HAWAII		
HONOLULU	Kapiolani-Children's Medical Center, 1319 Punahou Street, Honolulu, HI 96826	808 941-4411, 808 362-3585
IDAHO		
BOISE	Idaho Emergency Medical Poison Center, 1055 North Curtis Road, Boise, ID 83706	208 334-2241, 800 632-8000 (Statewide)
POCATELLO	Idaho Drug Information Service and Poison Control Center, Pocatello Regional Medical Ctr., 777 Hospital Way, Pocatello, ID 83202	208 234-0777 Ext. 2019, 800 632-9490 (Statewide)
ILLINOIS		
CHICAGO	Rush Presbyterian–St. Luke's Poison Center, Rush Presbyterian–St. Luke's Medical Center, 1753 West Congress Pkwy., Chicago, IL 60612	312 942-5969, 800 942-5969 (Chicago and N.E. Illinois)
PEORIA	Peoria Poison Center, St. Francis Hospital and Medical Center, 530 N. E. Glen Oak Avenue, Peoria, IL 61637	309 672-2334, 800 322-5330 (Northern & Central Illinois)

SPRINGFIELD	Central and Southern Illinois Poison Resource Center, St. John's Hospital, 800 E. Carpenter, Springfield, IL 62769	217 753-3330, 800 252-2022 (Statewide)

INDIANA

EVANSVILLE	Poison Control Center, Deaconess Hospital, Inc., 600 Mary Street, Evansville, IN 47710	812 426-3333
	Welborn Memorial Baptist Hospital, 401 S. E. 6th Street, Evansville, IN 47713	812 426-8336
FORT WAYNE	Emergency Department, Lutheran Hospital, 3024 Fairfield Avenue, Fort Wayne, IN 46807	219 458-2211
	Parkview Memorial Hospital, 2200 Randalia Drive, Fort Wayne, IN 46805	219 484-9711
GARY	Methodist Hospital of Gary, Ind., 600 Grant Street, Gary, IN 46402	219 886-4710
HAMMOND	Poison Control Center, St. Margaret's Hospital, 25 Douglas Street, Hammond, IN 46320	219 931-4477
INDIANAPOLIS	Indiana Poison Center, 1001 West Tenth Street, Indianapolis, IN 46202	317 630-7351, 800 382-9097
MUNCIE	Ball Memorial Hospital, 2401 University Avenue, Muncie, IN 47303	317 747-4321
SOUTH BEND	St. Joseph's Medical Center, 811 East Madison Street, South Bend, IN 46622	219 237-7264

IOWA

DES MOINES	Variety Club Poison & Drug Information Center, Iowa Methodist Medical Ctr., 1200 Pleasant Street, Des Moines, IA 50308	515 283-6254, 800 362-2327 (Statewide)
FORT DODGE	Trinity Regional Hospital, Kenyon Road, Fort Dodge, IA 50501	515 573-3101
IOWA CITY	University of Iowa Hospitals and Clinics, Poison Control Center, Iowa City, IA 52242	319 356-2922, 800 272-6477 (Statewide)

KANSAS

KANSAS CITY	Mid-American Poison Center, University of Kansas, 39th and Rainbow Blvd., Kansas City, KS 66103	913 588-6633, 800 332-6633 (Statewide)
LAWRENCE	Lawrence Memorial Hospital, 325 Maine Street, Lawrence, KS 66044	913 843-3680 Ext. 162
TOPEKA	Stormont–Vail Regional Medical Center, 10th & Washburn Streets, Topeka, KS 66606	913 354-6100
	Northeast Kansas Poison Ctr., St. Francis Hospital, 1700 West 7th Street, Topeka, KS 66606	913 295-8094
WICHITA	Wesley Medical Center, 550 N. Hillside Avenue, Wichita, KS 67214	316 688-2277

KENTUCKY

FORT THOMAS	St. Luke's Hospital, 85 North Grand Avenue, Fort Thomas, KY 41075	606 572-3215, 800 352-9900 (Statewide)
LEXINGTON	Central Baptist Hospital, 1740 S. Limestone Street, Lexington, KY 40503	606 278-3411 Ext. 363
	Drug Information Center, University of Kentucky Medical Center, Lexington, KY 40536	606 233-5320
LOUISVILLE	Kentucky Regional Poison Ctr. of Kosair–Children's Hospital NKC, INC, P. O. Box 35070, Louisville, KY 40232	502 589-8222, 800 722-5725 (Statewide)
PADUCAH	Western Baptist Hospital, 2501 Kentucky Avenue, Paducah, KY 42001	502 444-5180

LOUISIANA

MONROE	School of Pharmacy, Northeast Louisiana University, 700 University Avenue, Monroe, LA 71209	318 342-3008
	St. Francis Hospital, P. O. Box 1901, Monroe, LA 71301	318 325-6454
NEW ORLEANS	Charity Hospital, 1532 Tulane Avenue, New Orleans, LA 70140	504 568-5222
SHREVEPORT	Louisiana State University Poison Control and Drug Abuse Information Center, LSU Medical Center, P. O. Box 33932, Shreveport, LA 71130	318 425-1524

MAINE

PORTLAND
Maine Medical Center
Emergency Division
22 Bramhall Street
Portland, ME 04102
207 871-2381
800 442-6305 (Statewide)

MARYLAND

BALTIMORE
Maryland Poison Center
University of Maryland
School of Pharmacy
636 West Lombard Street
Baltimore, MD 21201
301 528-7701
800 492-2414 (Statewide)

CUMBERLAND
Tri-State Poison Center
Sacred Heart Hospital
900 Seton Drive
Cumberland, MD 21502
301 722-6677

MASSACHUSETTS

BOSTON
Massachusetts Poison Control System
300 Longwood Avenue
Boston, MA 02115
617 232-2120
800 682-9211 (Statewide)
617 277-3323 TTY (MA Only)

MICHIGAN

ANN ARBOR
Poison Control Center
University Hospital
1405 East Ann Street
Ann Arbor, MI 48104
313 764-7667

DETROIT
S. E. Regional Poison Center
Children's Hospital of Michigan
3901 Beaubien
Detroit, MI 48201
313 494-5711
800 572-1655 (Statewide)

FLINT
Poison Information Center
Hurley Medical Center
One Hurley Plaza
Flint, MI 48502
313 257-9111
800 572-5396 (Statewide)

GRAND RAPIDS
Western Michigan Regional Poison Center
1840 Wealthy, S.E.
Grand Rapids, MI 49506
616 774-7854
800 632-2727 (Statewide)

LANSING
St. Lawrence Hospital
1210 West Saginaw Street
Lansing, MI 48914
517 372-5112

MARQUETTE
Upper Peninsula Regional Poison Center
Marquette General Hospital
420 West Magnetic Drive
Marquette, MI 49855
906 228-9440
800 562-9781 (N. MI only)

SAGINAW
Saginaw Region Poison Center
Saginaw General Hospital
1447 North Harrison
Saginaw, MI 48602
517 755-1111

MINNESOTA

DULUTH
St. Luke's Hospital
Poison Control Center
915 East First Street
Duluth, MN 55805
218 726-5466

St. Mary's Hospital
407 East 3rd St.
Duluth, MN 55805
218 726-4500

MINNEAPOLIS
Hennepin Poison Center
Hennepin County Medical Ctr.
701 Park Avenue
Minneapolis, MN 55415
612 347-3141

ROCHESTER
Southeastern Minnesota Poison Control Center
St. Mary's Hospital
1216 Second Street, S. W.
Rochester, MN 55901
507 285-5123

ST. PAUL
Minnesota Poison Information Center
St. Paul-Ramsey Medical Ctr.
640 Jackson Street
St. Paul, MN 55101
612 221-2113

MISSISSIPPI

COLUMBIA
Marion County General Hospital
Sunrall Road
Brandon, MS 39429
601 736-6303 Ext. 1020

GREENWOOD
Greenwood–Leflore Hospital
River Road
Greenwood, MS 38930
601 459-2790

JACKSON
University Medical Center
2500 North State Street
Jackson, MS 39216
601 354-7660

UNIVERSITY
University of Mississippi
School of Pharmacy
Poison Information Center
University, MS 38677
601 234-1522

MISSOURI

COLUMBIA
University of Missouri
Hospital and Clinics
807 Stadium Road
Columbia, MO 65212
314 882-8091

KANSAS CITY
Children's Mercy Hospital
24th at Gillham Road
Kansas City, MO 64108
816 234-3000

ST. LOUIS
St. Louis Regional Poison Ctr.
Cardinal Glennon Memorial Hospital for Children
1465 South Grand Avenue
St. Louis, MO. 63104
314 772-5200

St. Louis Children's Hospital
500 S. Kingshighway
St. Louis, MO 63110
314 454-6099

MONTANA

HELENA
Montana Poison Control System
Cogswell Building
Helena, MT 59620
406 442-2480
800 525-5042

NEBRASKA

OMAHA
Mid-Plains Regional Poison Ctr.
Children's Memorial Hospital
8301 Dodge
Omaha, NE 68114
402 390-5400
800 642-9999 (Statewide)
800 228-9515 (surrounding states)

NEW YORK

BUFFALO
Western New York Poison Control Center
Children's Hospital of Buffalo
219 Bryant Street
Buffalo, NY 14222
716 878-7654

EAST MEADOW
Long Island Regional Poison Control Center
Nassau County Medical Center
2201 Hempstead Turnpike
East Meadow, NY 11554
516 542-2324
516 542-2323 (TTY)

NEW YORK CITY
New York City Poison Ctr.
Department of Health
Bureau of Laboratories
455 First Avenue
New York City, NY 10016
212 340-4494
212 764-7667

NYACK
Hudson Valley Poison Ctr.
Nyack Hospital
N. Midland Avenue
Nyack, NY 10960
914 353-1000

ROCHESTER
Finger Lakes Poison Ctr. LIFELINE
University of Rochester Medical Center
Rochester, NY 14642
716 275-5151
716 275-2700 (TTY)

UTICA
St. Luke's Memorial Hospital Center
P. O. Box 479
Utica, NY 13502
315 798-6200

NORTH CAROLINA

ASHEVILLE
Western North Carolina Poison Control Center
Memorial Mission Hospital
509 Biltmore Avenue
Asheville, NC 28801
704 255-4490

CHARLOTTE
Mercy Hospital
2001 Vail Avenue
Charlotte, NC 28207
704 379-5827

DURHAM
Duke University Medical Center Poison Control Center
P. O. Box 3007
Durham, NC 27710
919 684-8111

JACKSONVILLE
Onslow Memorial Hospital
Western Blvd.
Jacksonville, NC 28540
919 577-2555

WILMINGTON
New Hanover Memorial Hospital
2131 South 17th St.
Wilmington, NC 28401
919 343-7046

NORTH DAKOTA

BISMARCK
Bismarck Hospital
Emergency Department
300 North 7th Street
Bismarck, ND 58501
701 223-4357

FARGO
St. Luke's Poison Center
St. Luke's Hospitals
Fifth Street at Mills Ave.
Fargo, ND 58122
701 280-5575

MINOT
St. Joseph's Hospital
Third St. & Fourth Ave., S. E.
Minot, ND 58701
701 857-2553

OHIO

AKRON
Children's Hospital Medical Center of Akron
281 Locust Street
Akron, OH 44308
216 379-8562
800 362-9922

CINCINNATI
Drug Poison Information Ctr.
Bridge Medical Science Bldg.
Room 7701
231 Bethesda Avenue
Cincinnati, OH 45267
513 872-5111

CLEVELAND
Greater Cleveland Poison Control Center
2119 Abington Road
Cleveland, OH 44106
216 231-4455

COLUMBUS
Central Ohio Poison Center
Children's Hospital of Ohio
700 Children's Drive
Columbus, OH 43205
614 228-1323

DAYTON
Children's Medical Center
One Children's Plaza
Dayton, OH 45404
513 222-2227
800 762-0727 (Statewide)

OKLAHOMA

LAWTON
Comanche County Memorial Hospital
3401 Gore Blvd.
Lawton, OK 73501
405 355-8620

OKLAHOMA CITY
Oklahoma Poison Control Ctr.
Oklahoma Children's Memorial Center
P. O Box 26307
Oklahoma City, OK 73126
405 271-5454
800 522-4611

TULSA
Hillcrest Medical Center
1120 South Utica
Tulsa, OK 74104
918 560-5755

STATE COORDINATOR

OREGON
Oregon Poison Control and Drug Information Center
University of Oregon Health Sciences Center
Portland, OR 97201
503 225-8968
800 452-7165 (Statewide)

ANCON
PANAMA
U.S.A. MEDDAC Panama
Gorgas U.S. Army Hospital
Ancon, Panama
APO Miami 34004
507 252-7500

ALLENTOWN
PENNSYLVANIA
Lehigh Valley Poison Center
Allentown General Hospital
17th & Chew Streets
Allentown, PA 18102
215 433-2311

HERSHEY
Capital Area Poison Center
The Milton S. Hershey Medical Center
University Drive
Hershey, PA 17033
717 534-6111 (Treatment)

PHILADELPHIA
Philadelphia Poison Information
3211 University Avenue
Philadelphia, PA 19104
215 922-5523
922-5524

PITTSBURGH
Pittsburgh Poison Center
Children's Hospital
125 DeSoto Street
Pittsburgh, PA 15214
412 681-6669
647-5600

ARECIBO
PUERTO RICO
District Hospital of Arecibo
Arecibo, PR 00613
809 765-4880
765-0615

RIO PIEDRAS
Childrens Hospital Center of Puerto Rico
Rio Piedras, PR 00936
809 754-8535

SAN JUAN
Pharmacy School
Medical Sciences Campus
San Juan, PR 00936
809 753-4849

PROVIDENCE
RHODE ISLAND
Rhode Island Poison Center
Rhode Island Hospital
Annex Bldg. 422
593 Eddy Street
Providence, RI 02902
401 277-5727

CHARLESTON
SOUTH CAROLINA
National Pesticide Telecommunications Network
Medical University of South Carolina
171 Ashley Avenue
Charleston, SC 29403
803 792-4201
800 845-7633 (Outside SC)

COLUMBIA
Palmetto Poison Center
University of South Carolina
College of Pharmacy
Columbia, SC 29208
803 765-7359
800 922-1117

RAPID CITY
SOUTH DAKOTA
Rapid City Regional Poison Control Center
353 Fairmont Blvd.
P. O. Box 6000
Rapid City, SD 57709
605 341-3333
800 742-8925

SIOUX FALLS
McKennan Poison Center
McKennan Hospital
800 East 21st Street
Sioux Falls, SD 57101
605 336-3894
800 952-0123 (Statewide)

KNOXVILLE
TENNESSEE
Memorial Research Center Hospital
1924 Alcoa Hwy.
Knoxville, TN 37920
615 971-3261

MEMPHIS
Southern Poison Center
LeBonheur Children's Medical Center
848 Adams Avenue
Memphis, TN 38103
901 528-6048

NASHVILLE
Vanderbilt University Hospital
21st and Garland
Nashville, TN 37232
615 322-6435

EL PASO
TEXAS
El Paso Poison Control Center
R. E. Thomason General Hospital
4815 Alameda Avenue
El Paso, TX 79905
915 533-1244

FORT WORTH
W. I. Cook Children's Hospital
Cook Poison Center-Fort Worth
1212 West Lancaster Street
Fort Worth, TX 76102
817 336-6611

GALVESTON
Southeast Texas Poison Center
The University of Texas Medical Branch
Eighth & Mechanic Streets
Galveston, TX 77550
713 765-1420

HOUSTON
Southeast Texas Poison Control Center
Eighth & Mechanic Streets
Galveston, TX 77550
713 654-1701

SAN ANTONIO
Department of Pediatrics
University of Texas Health Science Center at San Antonio
7703 Floyd Curl Drive
San Antonio, TX 78284
512 223-6361 Ext. 473

WACO
Hillcrest Baptist Hospital
3000 Herring Avenue
Waco, TX 76708
817 753-1412

UTAH

SALT LAKE CITY	Intermountain Regional Poison Control Center, 50 North Medical Drive, Salt Lake City, UT 84132	801 581-2151

VERMONT

BURLINGTON	Vermont Poison Center, Medical Center Hospital of Vermont, Burlington, VT 05401	802 658-3456

VIRGINIA

CHARLOTTESVILLE	Blue Ridge Poison Center, University of Virginia Hospital, Charlottesville, VA 22903	804 924-5543, 800 446-9876 (TTY) (Out-of-state), 800 552-3723 (TTY) (Statewide)
NORFOLK	DePaul Hospital, Granby Street at Kingsley La., Norfolk, VA 23505	804 489-5288
RICHMOND	Central Virginia Poison Ctr. Medical College of Virginia, Virginia Commonwealth University, P. O. Box 522, MCV Station, Richmond, VA 23298	804 786-9123
ROANOKE	Southwest Virginia Poison Ctr. Roanoke Memorial Hospital, Belleview at Jefferson Street, P. O. Box 13367, Roanoke, VA 24033	703 981-7336

VIRGIN ISLANDS

ST. THOMAS	Knud-Hansen Memorial Hospital, St. Thomas, VI 00801	809 774-9000 Ext. 224/5, 809 774-1212

WASHINGTON

SEATTLE	Seattle Poison Center, Children's Orthopedic Hospital and Medical Ctr., 4800 Sand Point Way, NE, Seattle, WA 98105	206 634-5252, 800-732-6985
SPOKANE	Spokane Poison Center, Deaconess Hospital, West 800 Fifth Avenue, Spokane, WA 99210	509 747-1077, 800 572-5842 (Statewide), 509 747-1077 (TTY)
TACOMA	Mary Bridge Poison Information Center, Mary Bridge Children's Hospital, South L Street, Tacoma, WA 98405	206 272-1281

WEST VIRGINIA

STATE COORDINATOR	The West Virginia Poison System, West Virginia University School of Pharmacy, 3110 Mac Corkle Avenue, S. E., Charleston, WV 25304	304 348-4211

WISCONSIN

EAU CLAIRE	Eau Claire Poison Center, Luther Hospital, 1225 Whipple, Eau Claire, WI 54701	715 835-1515
MADISON	Madison Area Poison Center, University Hospital & Clinic, 600 Highland Avenue, Madison, WI 53792	608 262-3702
MILWAUKEE	Milwaukee Poison Center, Milwaukee Children's Hospital, 1700 West Wisconsin Avenue, Milwaukee, WI 53233	414 931-4114

WYOMING

CHEYENNE	Wyoming Poison Center, DePaul Hospital, 2600 East 18th Street, Cheyenne, WY 82001	307 635-9256, 800 442-2704

CHAPTER THREE

Poisons in Your Garden

Mary, Mary, quite contrary
How does your garden grow?
With silver bells and cockle shells
And poisons all in a row.

It's not a lie. According to scientific records, more than 700 types of plants in the northern hemisphere have caused illness or loss of life. Experts are also sure that many plants that have not yet been identified as poisonous really are.

The percentage of poisonous plants is not very high, but many are so beautiful, and so well known, that it is hard to believe they can be lethal. Poisonous plants can easily be found in your garden and foundation plantings as well as growing in vacant lots and woods. The U.S. Public Health Service reports that thousands of children eat potentially poisonous plants every year. However, as the Greater New York Safety Council has pointed out:

> There is no reason to stop growing beautiful flowers and plants because they contain poison, just keep them out of your mouth. Train children not to chew on anything other than known foods, no matter how familiar it appears to be.
>
> Keep a close watch on the little ones in the hand-to-mouth stage. Remember too, adults are not immune to unconscious nibbling.

Cherry, Peach Tree, and Other Dangers

Plants can be tricky. Often one part of a plant is not only edible, but nutritious, while another part can kill if it is eaten. Twigs of cherry trees release deadly cyanide when eaten and the leaves of peach trees contain one of the most dangerous poisons known, hydrocyanic acid. Children have become very ill after drinking a "tea" made with hot water and peach tree leaves.

Fruit trees aren't the only plant deceivers. Even such common vegetables as the potato, tomato and rhubarb can cause illness. Obviously, fresh tomatoes and potatoes are harmless, but the leaves and vines of both of these plants contain poisons that can cause severe stomach upsets and nervous disorders.

The rhubarb's delicious stalk is commonly used in cooking, yet it is the most dangerous plant in your vegetable garden. Rhubarb leaves contain oxalic acid which turns to crystals when it reaches the kidneys and causes severe damage.

Who would ever guess that the beautiful, flowering oleander bush contains a deadly heart stimulant? This poison is so powerful that a single leaf of oleander can kill a child. The plant is so deadly that a number of people have died just from eating steaks that were speared with oleander sticks and roasted over a fire. If you do use sticks to cook upon or with, be sure they are safe.

Do you have hyacinths, narcissus, or daffodils around the house? Poisons from their bulbs cause nausea, vomiting, and diarrhea, and may be fatal.

Rhododendron, azalea, daphne, and wisteria have leaves, stems and berries that can kill your child.

Larkspur, lily-of-the-valley, iris, pea, autumn crocus, and bleeding heart are a few more familiar plants which have poisonous flowers, stems, leaves, seeds, roots, berries, or bulbs.

There is enough poison in a tiny packet of castor beans to kill half-a-dozen youngsters. One rosary pea seed can kill a child. Beautiful holiday greens and plants are nice to have around, but mistletoe, holly, Jerusalem cherry, and poinsettia can all cause serious cases of poisoning. Some years ago a group of 30 boys returned from an outing with their orphanage in the Midwest. Within only a few hours after their return, the boys went wild. Some began to laugh hysterically, others barked like dogs, and some plucked imaginary objects out of the air. A visiting physician administered the proper drugs and induced vomiting in the boys. Their crazy antics came from eating jimson weed. Sometimes called thorn apple or stinkweed, this poison plant grows almost everywhere. It is responsible for more poisonings than any other plant. Its large, white, funnel-type flowers resemble morning glories. The plant has large leaves and grows from two to five feet tall. All parts of the jimson weed are poisonous, but its seeds and leaves are especially dangerous.

Beware the Hemlock

Socrates was put to death by being forced to drink a brew made from poison hemlock, a common plant with lacy foliage that grows in clumps and has a rounded, carrot-like projection. The deadly hemlock, in fact, resembles the wild carrot and is a member of the carrot family. It has many other killer relatives.

How many parents know, for example, that the yews, common garden evergreens used in rock gardens and foundation plantings, are also a type of hemlock and that poisons abound in both its needle-like leaves and colorful berries? In fact, other hedge plants, such as the box, privet, and hydrangea, are all dangerous if leaf clippings or small plants are eaten.

As for wild mushrooms, the best rule is to leave them to the experts. Most of them—no matter how much they look like the kind of mushrooms you buy in the store—are poisonous. **Don't pick and eat wild mushrooms unless you are an expert in mushroom identification.**

In his book, *Deadly Harvest*, Dr. John Kingsbury gives this advice concerning poisonous plants:

1. Learn the poisonous plants in your neighborhood.

2. Take as a firm rule, and impress upon children,

never to eat any unknown garden or wild plant, herb, shrub, or tree; never to make medical preparations from them. Also keep dangerous prunings, clippings, or garden cleanings away from livestock.

3. In any case of poisoning or suspected poisoning, call your physician, and be prepared, if at all possible, to tell him the name of the plant involved. Save evidence which might help identify the plant. Such evidence includes plant parts taken from the mouth or present in vomit or stools.

Leaves of Three, Let Them Be

While you may not have been aware of the dangers of the plants and flowers we have discussed, there is one group of poisonous plants with which you are certainly familiar. These are poison ivy, poison oak, and poison sumac.

Whatever you do, do no believe the old wives' tale that chewing the leaves of these plants will make you immune to the rashes they cause. You may not live if you try it.

Learn to recognize these dangerous plants from the drawings of them on these pages. **Then keep your family away from them.**

If a family member does come in contact with any of the three, he or she will probably develop a skin rash that will begin as small, itchy bumps and eventually turn to small blisters.

After contact with poison ivy, oak, or sumac:

✔ Remove clothes that have come in contact with the plants and wash them in strong laundry soap before using them again. Be careful not to touch the contaminated area yourself.

✔ Immediately wash the skin that came in contact with the plants with a strong laundry soap.

✔ You may use calamine lotion to ease itching.

✔ Do not let the child scratch and spread the rash.

✔ Watch for severe allergic reactions (see page 56) and call a doctor or a hospital immediately if you note them.

✔ If the rash covers a large portion of the body, or grows continually more severe and uncomfortable, seek medical help as soon as possible.

✔ Be careful to avoid the fumes of burning poison ivy, oak and sumac. These can be extremely irritating to the lungs.

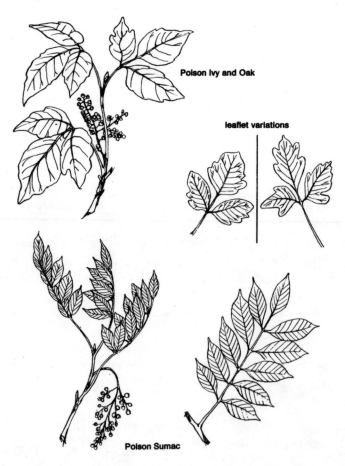

Poison Ivy and Oak

leaflet variations

Poison Sumac

More Poisonous Plants

Here is a list of some other common, poisonous plants. When a child eats a plant not listed, or one you cannot identify, follow the instructions on page 14.

House and Garden Plants

Autumn crocus. Bulbs are poisonous.

Castor bean and rosary pea. All parts are poisonous. One or two of either of these seeds can kill a child.

Dumb cane (dieffenbachia). All parts are poisonous. Causes severe burning of mouth and tongue.

Hyacinth, Narcissus, Daffodil. Bulbs are poisonous.

Iris. Leaves and roots are poisonous.

Lily of the Valley. All parts are poisonous.

Oleander. Leaves and branches are poisonous.

Poinsettia. Juice of leaves, stems and flowers, as well as the fruit, are poisonous.

Vegetable Garden Plants

Potato. Leaves and vines, as well as the green spots or potato tubers, are poisonous.

Rhubarb. Leaf blades are poisonous.

Tomato. Leaves and vines are poisonous.

Trees and Shrubs

Cherry and peach. Leaves and twigs are poisonous.

Laurel, Rhododendron, Azalea. All parts are poisonous.

Oaks. Acorns and leaves are poisonous. The symptoms appear only after eating these parts for a period of time. Do not allow children to chew acorns.

Yews. Berries and leaves are poisonous.

Wild Plants and Flowers

Buttercup. All parts are poisonous.

Jimson weed or thorn apple. All parts are poisonous, especially the seeds.

Nightshade. All parts are poisonous, especially the unripe berry.

May apple. Green apple, leaves, roots are poisonous.

Mushrooms (wild). All parts may be poisonous.

Poison Hemlock. The leaves, stem and fruit of this plant, which resembles large wild carrot, are poisonous.

What to Do

If a child eats a part of a plant that you suspect is poisonous:

1. Call the Poison Control Center or the doctor or hospital immediately. Give them all the information you have about the poison and the child. Write down and follow their directions.

2. If you cannot reach any of the above, don't waste any more time trying. If another person is available, let him do the calling while you DILUTE THE POISON. Do this by giving the child a glass of milk or water.

3. Make the child vomit if so directed, but not if the child is unconscious or having fits. (See directions for making a child vomit on page 16). Do not waste time waiting for the child to vomit if he does not do so right away. Take the child to a doctor or hospital emergency room right away. Bring any parts of the plant the child may have eaten for identification.

If the child has stopped breathing, administer mouth-to-mouth breathing and external heart massage if necessary. (See pages 4 and 6.)

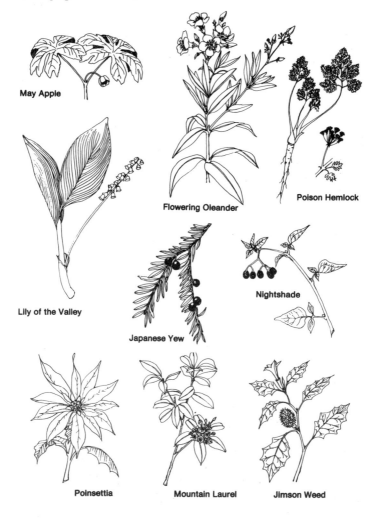

May Apple

Flowering Oleander

Poison Hemlock

Lily of the Valley

Japanese Yew

Nightshade

Poinsettia

Mountain Laurel

Jimson Weed

CHAPTER FOUR

Accident-Proof Your Home

Your home may be a death trap for your children. Accidents kill more children between the ages of 1 and 14 than any disease.

Here are some of the frightening statistics, shown for the latest years available.

DEATHS FROM ACCIDENTS AND DISEASE 1-14 YEARS, 1980

8,337—ALL Accidents
3,926—Motor Vehicle Accidents
3,337—Home Accidents
2,070—Cancer
1,587—Congenital Anomalies

ALL ACCIDENTAL DEATHS* IN 1983 OF CHILDREN UNDER 15

Total.. 8,700
Motor Vehicle... 3,700
Fires, burns & deaths associated with fires.............. 1,050
Falls 350
Firearms.. 260
Poisons (solid and liquid)............................... 110
Poisonous gas 80
Suffocation—ingested object 250
All other types 1,350

*Approximations by National Safety Council based on data from National Center for Health Statistics, state health departments, and city and state traffic authorities.

Those statistics add up to some pretty frightening numbers. Home accidents that cause injuries that do not kill, but require hospital treatment, are even more common, and exceed half a million each year. If there are dangers in and around your home, and you do not take the time to correct them, you may be endangering your child's life.

Here is a room-by-room checklist of things you must correct if you wish to cut the chances of accidents involving children in your home.

General Checklist

✔ Keep cigarettes, tobacco, and ashtrays out of the reach of children. The tobacco from one cigarette, if eaten, can kill a young child. Be sure you have enough ashtrays to prevent the ashes from being flicked onto the floor or furniture where they can start fires.

✔ Be certain that all of your rugs and carpets are secured. Are there any frayed or loose edges that can cause trips and falls?

✔ Check all the cords on your electrical appliances and lights. Be sure they are not frayed. If they are, it is an easy matter to repair them.

✔ Don't overload sockets in the wall or on extension cords. Overloaded electrical outlets can cause fires.

✔ Never replace a burnt-out fuse with a penny. Use only another fuse that is the correct size. A fuse is a safety item, designed to blow if its circuit is overloaded. If the fuse is too big, or if you use a penny or a slug, the wiring in your home can become overloaded, grow dangerously hot, and start fires.

✔ Repair all peeling paint or falling plaster. Falling plaster can cause concussions in small children, and they may choke on bits of it. Peeling lead-based paint, if eaten, can cause lead poisoning.

✔ Be careful with your television set. It can kill. Competent servicemen can eliminate hazards. Don't attempt to fix your TV set unless you are an expert. Electricity in a television set may run higher than 20,000 volts, and that electricity strives to get the shortest route to the ground. You can provide that route through proper grounding. Make sure your set is well ventilated, for it can get very hot and catch fire.

Implosion is the most feared television set accident. This can happen when a picture tube—which is under very high pressure—is damaged or jarred. The glass is sucked inward slowly and then shoots out, spraying sharp pieces of glass many feet. Get rid of old picture tubes immediately.

✔ Check your outside antenna. Is it mounted properly? Does your house have a lightning rod?

✔ Don't leave dishes of nuts, small candies or other snacks where youngsters can reach them. These objects can easily choke and kill a child.

✔ If you have any large glass sliding doors or picture windows, mark them with paint, tape, or decals. A child or stranger in your home could easily walk through such a sheet of glass and cause a serious injury.

✔ Are any steps slippery or in disrepair? If they are, they should be repaired quickly. Is the carpeting on steps frayed or loose?

✔ Don't fix any electrical equipment or appliance if you aren't familiar with it. You may electrocute yourself or make an error that could cause a fire or burns at a later time.

✔ Do you have banisters or guard rails near your steps? Are they loose or in other disrepair? If so, fix them.

✔ You should have guard rails across any windows that a child might be able to reach. Children frequently fall out of windows and seriously injure themselves. However, window protection devices should be removable from *the outside* in case of fire or other emergency.

✔ Do you have guard gates in front of any steps or drop-offs where a child might venture? Be sure that you remove these gates as soon as a child is able to climb, or a more serious accident could result.

✔ Do you have any bookcases or other furniture that a child might be able to pull over onto himself or herself? Could the child pull something from shelves or pull a carpet out from under a piece of furniture and be injured by the falling object?

✔ Has your family planned the escape routes they will take in case of fire?

✔ If you have bolts that lock with keys from the inside of the house as well as from the outside, be sure that every member of the family knows where the keys are. If you do not do this, your family might be unable to escape a fire.

✔ Dispose of all aerosol cans properly. Keep them out of the reach of children at all times.

✔ Do not use thin plastic film or plastic cleaners' bags to cover furniture. This type of material can suffocate a child in only a few moments.

✔ Are there any exposed radiators or steam pipes in reach of a child? If so, these should be covered with insulation. Children have received severe burns on their hands from grabbing or touching hot pipes.

✔ Fireworks or firecrackers are dangerous items that should be banned from your home. Most communities have July 4th firework shows supervised by the local fire department. Such shows are more beautiful, and much safer, than any you could put on at home.

✔ Are all rooms, halls, and stairs well lit to avoid trips and falls?

✔ Is all furniture placed so it does not block halls or doorways?

✔ Don't smoke in bed—ever!

✔ Never use candles or matches to search in dark closets or closed areas.

✔ Throw away all old papers, rags, and other materials that burn easily.

✔ Cover all unused electrical outlets with plastic plugs made especially for this purpose. A child can be electrocuted by poking keys, pins, or other small metal objects into electrical outlets.

✔ Inspect your neighborhood for dangers. Are there any open wells or sewers? Are there any vacant lots with dangerous rubbish? Are there any weak or broken electrical poles or wiring? Any unsafe intersections? If you find these or other dangers lurking near your home, get together with concerned neighbors and take the matter up with local authorities. If they can't help you, find out who is responsible; your local newspaper should be able to help.

Kitchen Checklist

More than 150,000 people receive hospital emergency room treatment each year for injuries associated with kitchen knives or ranges.

✔ When you are cooking, do you keep your pan and pot handles turned away from the front of the range? A child could easily reach up to the stove and pour boiling liquids all over his or her body.

✔ Can your child reach the range controls to turn on the gas? If he or she can, there is danger. Many people prefer to remove the knobs from their stove when they are not cooking. This is only a small inconvenience compared with a possible death from gas fumes.

✔ Be sure to keep dangerous chemicals or cleaning products away from the cabinet beneath the kitchen sink, or keep the cabinet locked. Even vanilla and almond food extracts are poisonous if they are taken straight from the bottle.

✔ Don't keep foods and cleaning chemicals together in the same pantry. Mixups can be fatal.

✔ Be sure that tables, chairs, and especially high chairs are stable and cannot fall on a child or tip over when a child is sitting in them.

✔ Don't leave bottles, plates, or serving platters on the edge of a counter where a child can reach up, grab them, and pull them down onto herself or himself.

✔ Follow operating and safety instructions for microwave ovens. Never operate if door does not close firmly. Do not stand against a microwave oven, or allow children to, for long periods of time when it is operating.

✔ Store matches in a fireproof container that you keep out of children's reach.

✔ Never keep the toaster, blender, or can opener in a location where a child could grab the cord and pull these appliances on top of herself or himself.

✔ Are all electrical plugs and connections out of a child's reach?

✔ Do you have a fire extinguisher in your kitchen? Get one! In case of a fire, if an extinguisher is not available, never pour water on an oil or grease fire. Use baking soda to smother the flames. Call the fire department.

✔ Never leave your child alone in the kitchen. He or she could choke on a piece of food as "harmless" as a cracker or cookie.

✔ Keep knives, scissors, and other dangerous utensils in places where your child cannot reach them.

Bathroom Checklist

Some 200 drownings and 200,000 nonfatal bathroom injuries occur in the United States every year.

✔ Do you have bathmats, safety tapes, or rubber appliques on the floor of the shower or tub? Slips and falls can cause serious injury to adults as well as children.

✔ Is the rod for your shower curtain secure enough so it cannot fall onto a small head?

✔ All bathroom cabinets must be locked or out of a child's reach. Remember that youngsters can climb.

✔ Clean out medicine cabinets. Throw away all old and unlabeled medicines. Make sure all of your future prescriptions are labeled. Request this service from your doctor and pharmacist.

✔ Rugs or mats on your bathroom floor should be secure. Many kinds of bathroom rugs are available with no-skid or rubber bottoms.

✔ Are all radios, electric razors, and other electrical appliances out of the reach of any person taking a bath? Turning a radio off or on, or shaving with an electric razor in the bath are dangerous. Buy appliances with the Underwriters Laboratories (UL) label.

✔ Install ground fault circuit interrupters (GFCI) in new and remodeled bathrooms. The GFCI prevents electric shock from faulty equipment by monitoring and interrupting electricity flow.

✔ Do you have a safety rail or grab bar in your bathtub?

✔ Remove glass bottles or jars from the top of the toilet tank and those in and around the tub. Almost all shampoos, soaps, or bath oils are available in nonbreakable plastic containers.

✔ Never leave razors—electric or safety—lying around.

Always dispose of blades in receptacles provided or in another safe place.

✔ No glass drinking glasses should be allowed in the bathroom. Plastic or disposable paper cups are the safe way.

✔ When you give a baby or small child a bath, NEVER leave the child so you can answer the phone or doorbell or for any other reason. If the caller has something important to say, he will call back. Your child could drown quickly in as little as one inch of water.

✔ Always be on the lookout for slippery bathroom floors.

✔ Electric space heaters must not be allowed in the bathroom.

✔ Teach the child to use faucets properly as soon as he or she is able. The child could easily be scalded if he or she is not familiar with their use.

✔ Give all medications yourself. Make sure you read the label TWICE before administering medications, and make sure that you are wide awake when doing so. If you give medicine to a child in the middle of the night, you will be wise to jot down a note on what you gave the child. This way there can be no confusion or forgetting in the morning.

Nursery Checklist

✔ Don't buy a crib with the side slats too far apart. Your child could get his or her head caught between them and be strangled. Plastic or rubber bumper rails are available for almost all crib sizes.

✔ Check the room to eliminate peeling paint or falling plaster.

✔ Always use nontoxic paint to paint a child's room and furniture.

✔ Never leave a baby unattended on a bassinet or table.

✔ Don't use the crib as a playpen.

✔ Never leave a baby unattended when the side of the crib is down.

✔ Never use plastic bags as sheet covers in your child's bed. They may save you from washing one set of sheets, but there is a good chance plastic bags will suffocate and kill your child. Safe, moisture-proof pads are available at most department stores.

✔ Check and repair or eliminate any furniture that might be able to tip over onto a child.

✔ Periodically check all of the nuts, bolts, and screws on your child's crib. These loosen because of the child's movement. If not tightened, the crib could collapse and injure or kill your baby.

✔ Keep toys in their own special place. Don't let them remain strewn about the room to trip and injure someone. Teach your child to be tidy and put things away.

✔ Make sure that vaporizers and other appliances are safely located.

✔ Make sure all rugs have nonskid backing.

✔ Don't buy your child dangerous toys. Choose them carefully. (See Chapter 10.)

Attic, Basement, Garage, and Shed Checklist

The National Safety Council says that after kitchens, these are the most dangerous areas of your home. **First of all, these areas should be off-limits for your small children. There are simply too many dangers. You should also follow these precautions:**

✔ All tools must be stored away from curious children.

✔ Lawn equipment should be stored safely. Always store rakes, hoes, and shovels with the tines or blades down, or hang them on the wall with the sharp sides facing inward.

✔ All chemical fertilizers, pesticides, and paint removers should be labeled properly and stored well out of reach or in locked cabinets.

✔ Ropes, cords, and hoses must be out of reach. A child can be accidentally strangled or hanged.

✔ Throw away all plastic bags or tarpaulins. A child can suffocate in them.

✔ Close and lock, or remove the lids and doors of all trunks, big boxes, old refrigerators, or freezers. A child can get trapped inside and suffocate.

✔ Lock up or dispose of properly all guns, knives, swords, and other sharp objects.

✔ Get rid of all broken glass and mirrors.

✔ Get rid of all sharp, splintered wood, or wood with nails protruding.

✔ Make sure your attic, basement, garage, and sheds are properly illuminated.

✔ Keep children away from washers, dryers, and heating units.

✔ Never run your car, lawn mower, or other internal combustion engines in a closed garage or room. The fumes can kill.

✔ Don't let children use power tools. Disconnect them when they are not in use.

✔ Keep attics, basement, and garages orderly and free of debris.

✔ Teach children how to use sharp objects, cutting away from themselves. And teach them how to pass cutting or pointed objects to another person, handle first.

Pool, Patio, and Garden Checklist

✔ Forbid use of portable electric appliances within 10 feet of the pool.

✔ Keep extension cords away from poolside.

✔ Take care in handling poolside accessories. Handling things while you are wet can cause shocks.

✔ Be aware of the danger spots in a pool's wiring. These include filter pump motor, filter, time clock, pool cleaning equipment, electrically operated pool covers, and heating equipment.

✔ No glass should be allowed in the pool area. Use plastic or paper cups, plates, or pitchers.

✔ Be sure your pool area is properly fenced. Dozens of children die each year from drowning in unfenced backyard pools.

✔ No children should ever be allowed to swim alone. The "buddy system" used in many camps is an effective way of preventing accidents. The "buddy system" should be used *in addition to* adult supervision.

✔ No children should ever be allowed to swim when overtired, overheated, or just after eating.

✔ Discourage horseplay in the pool and patio area.

✔ Be sure you have the proper life preserving equipment in and around your pool

✔ Play it safe in barbecuing. Keep children away. Use gloves or potholders.

✔ If your house has a raised deck, be sure that its sides are safe and youngsters cannot fall through or over them.

✔ Do not overload decks. They can, and have, collapsed, resulting in tragic loss of lives.

✔ All outdoor electrical wiring and lighting should be done by an expert. It is too easy to get electrocuted from an amateur job.

✔ Make sure guests and children are aware of any poisonous plants or dangerous animals in or around your home.

✔ Make sure that playground equipment is safe and sturdy. No sharp edges or rust allowed.

*   *   *   *   *   *

Go through your entire house or apartment room by room, noting the corrections that need to be made. There may be some obvious ones that are not listed above. Now that you have found the potential dangers, eliminate them. You'll sleep better tonight when you are finished with this job.

First Aid Kit

You should make it a point to keep a well stocked first aid kit or box somewhere in your home. It should contain these essential items:

For covering open wounds and burns:
- sterile gauze squares
- sterile first aid dressing

For holding dressings:
- assorted gauze bandage
- roll adhesive tape

For cuts and scratches:
- assorted small adhesive bandages
- antibacterial soap

Miscellaneous:

- blunt-tip scissors
- tweezers
- aspirin or acetaminophen
- baby aspirin or baby dosage of acetaminophen
- thermometer
- cloth (for sling or tourniquet)
- flashlight
- paper cups for drinking
- table salt (small package)
- snakebite kit (optional, depending on where you live)
- essential personal prescriptions
- Syrup of Ipecac
- list of specific allergy problems in household
- list of phone numbers of physician, police, hospital,
- poison control center
- first aid book

CHAPTER FIVE

Burns and Electrical Injuries

Health and safety officials say that there are more than 2 million serious burn injuries in Canada and the United States every year. Many of these occur among children. In 1983 alone, more than 1,000 children were killed by fires and burns. Hundreds of thousands more were injured.

According to the American Academy of Pediatrics, the major causes of fire and burn accidents are:

- Defective electrical wiring and dangling cords.

- Improper storage of flammable materials.

- Adults who smoke in bed or dispose of cigarette ashes or butts improperly.

- Defective heating equipment.

- Overturned containers filled with hot food or water.

- Electrical appliances pulled by their cords.

- Dangerously flammable clothes.

All of the above can be corrected or eliminated. Most injuries due to fires and burns can be prevented, especially those that occur in the home. Practice fire drills with your family, and make sure you have one or more fire extinguishers placed strategically around your home.

Buy Safe Clothing

Safety studies indicate that nearly half of all fire deaths occur because clothing catches fire. Often the cause is the design of the clothing, such as flowing skirts or puffy sleeves.

You can eliminate many clothing-burn hazards by carefully selecting your child's wardrobe.

The selection of plain styles makes clothing safer, especially for little girls and women. (More girls than boys are involved in clothing fires because skirts and dresses hang away from the body and catch fire more easily.)

Even though almost all clothing will burn, some materials are safer than others. Here is a checklist, from the Michigan Department of Public Health, that will help you choose the safest possible fabric for your children's clothes.

NATURAL FIBERS

✔ **Wool.** This is the least flammable of all natural fibers. It is considered almost flame resistant in its natural state. When it catches fire, it will burn slowly and soon go out by itself.

✔ **Silk.** Silk alone is not very flammable, but it is often made more flammable by adding other materials to alter the color or texture.

✔ **Cotton.** This most commonly used cloth is highly flammable. It can, however, be made flame-retardant. (You can flame retard cotton fabrics by soaking them in a mixture of two quarts of warm water, seven ounces of borax and three ounces of boric acid. Drip dry and iron. Repeat process after each washing. KEEP CHILDREN AWAY FROM THE FIRE RETARDING MIXTURE.)

✔ **Linen.** This fabric is also quite flammable, but can be made flame-retardant in the same way as cotton.

✔ **Paper.** Paper clothes, too, are flammable, but can be made flame-retardant in the same way as cotton.

SYNTHETIC

✓ **Rayon, acetate, triacetate, etc.** These fibers are just as flammable as cotton, but can also be made flame-retardant in the same way as cotton.

✓ **Nylon, polyester, acrylic, etc.** These are often used in home furnishings because of their durability. Most of them are moderately flammable, and once ignited they offer added danger because they may melt and drip.

✓ **Textile glass fibers.** These are naturally flame-retardant.

The weight and weave of a fabric also helps to determine how fast it will ignite and burn. Tightly woven, heavy fabrics burn more slowly than loosely woven light fabrics of the same material.

Fortunately, in the area of safe clothes, the future looks promising. Industry has made progress in the use of safe and durable flame-retardant fabrics.

We can help increase the amount of flame-retardant clothing available by:

- Using flame-retardant materials now available.

- Creating a demand for more flame-retardant materials by asking for them at your local department or dry goods store.

United States law requires that all clothing bear a tag showing what it is made from. Look for these tags, which will help you buy safe clothing for your children.

Remember, although an article of clothing may be flame-retardant, *it is not flame proof.*

"Merry Christmas"

Have a merry Christmas. Don't buy a Christmas tree that will burn easily. Look for freshly cut trees that are not dried out. You can test this by trying to snap off a twig. If it snaps instead of bending, the tree is too dry. If too many needles fall to the ground when the tree is jarred, it is also too dry.

You can eliminate this difficulty by buying an artificial tree, but BE SURE YOU BUY ONE THAT IS FLAME-RETAR-DANT. Such trees can be used year after year.

Fresh trees can also be treated with fire retardants. Look for one that has been.

If you use a fresh tree, keep these suggestions in mind:

✔ Keep the cut stump moist at all times. This will retard the drying process.

✔ Do not keep your Christmas tree too long. The longer it stands in your home, the greater hazard it becomes.

✔ Brace the tree to be sure it will not fall over.

✔ Do not place the tree near heat sources.

✔ Use flame-retardant tree decorations.

✔ Use UL-approved lights for your tree, and be sure they are in good condition.

✔ Never overload electrical circuits.

To help prevent fires and burns in your home you should follow all of the general safety rules outlined in Chapter 4. NEVER LET CHILDREN PLAY WITH MATCHES OR LIGHTERS.

First Aid for Burns

There are several types of burns, but treatment for all of these types must include, in this order:

1. Prevention of shock (See Chapter 6).

2. Prevention of contamination.

3. Control of pain.

Never underestimate the severity of a burn. Burns are usually larger and more severe than you think.

In the case of burns from fire, here is what to do:

1. Get the child out of the burning area. If his or her clothes are on fire, do not let the child run. This will fan and encourage the flames. Put the fire out by wrapping the child in a blanket, rug, or other heavy material at hand.

2. If the burn is minor, immerse it in clean ice water, or apply ice packs to the area. (Wrap the ice in cloth or a towel.) Keep the burn area cold for at least 10 to 15 minutes. Cover the burn with a dressing, or a thin, no-stick plastic covering (clean plastic kitchen wrap works very well). Consult a physician.

IF THE BURN IS MORE SERIOUS:

1. Keep the child lying down. Try to keep the head and chest slightly lower than the rest of the body. Keep the child warm.

2. If the child is conscious and can swallow, give him nonalcoholic liquids to drink.

3. Keep watching for shock and treat if necessary.

4. Take the child to a doctor hospital immediately.

Important: Do not use butter, grease, ointments, or powders on burns. These increase the danger of infection and make treatment more difficult later.

Electrical Burns

If the child is still touching a source of electricity, you must get the child away from it. Do not touch the child's skin or you may also be electrocuted. Pull the child away by grabbing the dry clothing or use nonconductive material, such as heavy cloth, wood, or plastic to pull or pry the child from the electricity source.

Watch for signs of shock. If the child is not conscious, check the breathing and heart beat. If necessary, apply mouth-to-mouth breathing and external cardiac massage at once. (See pages 4 and 6.)

Contact the doctor, hospital, or police at once. If you are the only person available, however, continue mouth-to-mouth breathing and heart massage. Do not interrupt these procedures until:

- **The child is pronounced dead by a physician, or**
- **The child begins breathing normally again, or**
- **More than four hours pass without success.**

Chemical Burns

If you know what substance has caused these burns read the label on the container. It will give first aid measures. If this is not available:

1. Rinse the skin with lots of clean, cool water. Continue for at least five minutes. Use soap if possible.

2. Remove contaminated clothes.

3. Call the doctor, hospital, or police and get the patient to a hospital.

Chemicals in the Eyes

1. Immediately wash the eyes gently, with clean, cool water, with the eyelids open. Continue for at least five minutes. (Wash with milk if no clean water is available.)

2. Never let the child rub his or her eyes.

3. Remove contact lenses if they are being worn.

4. Call the doctor, hospital, or police and get the patient to a hospital.

CHAPTER SIX

How To Treat Shock

Shock is a complication that frequently accompanies other injuries, especially in children. It can be caused by a blow on the head, a broken bone, severe bleeding, poisoning, burns, electrical shock, or any number of other injuries.

It may also be caused by severe allergic reactions to animal or insect bites or stings, medicine, or poisonous plants. Any person with known allergies to medicines or other substances should wear a bracelet or necklace with a warning. Special jewelry is available from your doctor or druggist.

Basically, shock occurs because of an interruption in the flow of blood to the major organs such as the heart, brain, or kidneys.

In the case of an accident or injury, be on the lookout for shock.

Often shock may be more severe than the injury that brought it on. Shock can cause death. Whenever you give first aid treatment, be prepared to administer first aid for shock.

Symptoms of shock

The symptoms of shock include:

Cold, clammy skin

Faintness and lightheadedness

Rapid weak pulse

Irregular breathing
Paleness
Chills

What to Do

If these symptoms occur, treat the child in this manner:

1. **If possible, correct the cause.** (Stop bleeding, etc.)

2. **Keep the child lying down.** If possible, lower his head and chest below the rest of the body. At the very least, keep him lying flat. (This assures a good blood supply to the brain.)

3. **Keep breathing passages open.** Allow for plenty of fresh air.

4. **Keep the child warm with blankets or clothing.**

5. **If the child is conscious (and there is no injury to the abdominal area) you may let him drink warm, nonalcoholic fluids.**

6. **Call a physician, police or hospital.**

7. **Keep the child still and calm.**

Remember, shock can be more dangerous than the original injury. Be prepared to treat it.
You will know what you are doing, if you carefully read this book. Take control of the situation. Don't panic. Your confidence will be transferred to the child and will help his condition.

Insect, Spider, Snake and Animal Bites

Insect and spider stings are not usually dangerous, even though they frequently are painful or uncomfortable. There are, however, three circumstances in which an insect bite becomes an emergency situation.

The first of these situations arises if the guilty creature is a black widow spider, brown recluse spider or scorpion.

The famous *black widow* is shiny and, of course, black. It is usually about a half inch long and is easily recognized by the reddish hourglass marking on the spider's abdomen. The black widow is found in every state and usually lives outside the house under logs and old boards.

The *brown recluse* spider is about three quarters of an inch long and ranges in color from yellow to brown. This spider was once found only in the South and Midwest, but now can be found from coast to coast. The brown recluse can be identified by the violin or fiddle marking across its head and back. Because of this marking, the recluse is often called the fiddleback. It lives in the house in dark corners and closets, shoes, bedding, and clothes.

The *scorpion* is an animal that easily can be identified. It is black or dark brown, has four pairs of walking legs and a pair of strong pincers at the front of its body. Its tail is jointed and usually curled up. At the end of this tail is a stinger. Scorpions range in size from two to three inches. They are mainly nocturnal and can be found in the southern and western states. Scorpions will usually be found in a cool, dark place—under a stone or old, rusted can, or in a shoe, for example.

What to Do—Scorpions and poisonous spiders

If your child is bitten by a poisonous spider or scorpion, it is an emergency situation. Here is what to do:

1. Keep breathing passages open. Allow for plenty of fresh air. Restore breathing if necessary (see page 4).

2. Keep the bitten area lower than the victim's heart. Keep the child still.

3. Apply cold packs or ice packs wrapped in cloth to wound area.

4. Call a doctor or an ambulance, or carry child to emergency room. Do not—repeat—do not let the child walk.

The second circumstance under which an insect bite is an emergency is when a child receives multiple stings from a swarm of bees or wasps. Keep the child lying down, call a doctor, police, or a hospital.

The third circumstance under which an insect or spider bite is an emergency is when the bitten child develops signs of allergic reaction. These signs may include shortness of breath, wheezing, dizziness, headache, hives, runny nose, or nausea. If a child shows any indication of developing any of these signs after an insect or spider bite, keep the child calm and call the emergency room.

Watch for shock in all of the above situations. (See page 53.)

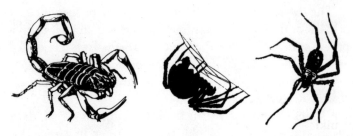

Scorpion (2 to 3 inches)   Black Widow (½-inch)   Brown Recluse (¾-inch)

What to Do—Bees and other stings

If your child receives a commonplace insect or spider bite or sting, and an emergency situation does not develop, here is what to do:

1. Remove the stinger, if there is one, by gently scraping with the edge of a clean knife blade or similar object. DO NOT USE A PAIR OF TWEEZERS, since this can squeeze the poison sac and cause even more poison to enter the body.

2. Wash the bite with plenty of soap and water.

3. Apply ice-cold compresses (but keep ice from direct contact with skin).

4. If pain persists, or any allergic reaction develops, call a physician immediately.

5. Calamine lotion or a thick baking soda and water paste will help relieve discomfort.

Animal Bites

Most animal bites do not cause serious problems other than the actual tissue damage inflicted. In the case of an animal bite, as for any dirty wound, you should contact your physician as soon as possible. He will probably want to check for infection and administer a tetanus inoculation to your child. This precaution is needed even in the case of bites by beloved household pets.

Animal bites are worrisome mainly because of the fear of rabies. Rabies is a viral disease, in which the virus attacks the brain and nervous system. Rabies was always fatal until 1971, when doctors pulled 7-year-old Matthew Winkler through a case of rabies he had contracted from a bat. But in all of medical history up to now, the case of Matthew Winkler is the single exception. Rabies is almost always fatal.

Fortunately, however, rabies takes a number of days to develop after a child is bitten by a rabid animal. So if your child has been infected, doctors can begin a series of treatments that will save his or her life. This treatment is quite painful, though, and should be avoided whenever possible.

The way to avoid it, of course, is for you to be on the lookout for bats, skunks, raccoons, foxes, or other wild animals in your neighborhood. These are the animals that frequently carry rabies, and the disease has been spreading among wild animals in recent years.

Rabies is also a possibility in the case of rat bites, the number of which seems to be steadily increasing in our urban areas. The bite of a rat should be treated just as the bite of any other potentially rabid animal.

It is difficult to identify a rabid animal if you are not an expert, so don't rely on being able to spot one. Instead, warn your child to stay away from all strange dogs, cats, or other animals, no matter how friendly they seem. Rabid animals often appear weak or dazed and helpless. Don't let your child be fooled. A normal wild animal will almost never approach a human; rabid wild animals do.

If your child is bitten by an animal:

1. Try to catch the animal that bit him. Call the police for assistance. Be sure not to take the chance of getting bitten yourself, but do not kill the animal unless you must. If you do have to kill it, try not to injure the animal's brain because this is the part of the dead animal that must be analyzed to determine whether or not rabies is present.

2. Wash the bite with lots of soap and water. Rinse it with clean water for two or three minutes. Cover with a sterile dressing.

3. Watch for signs of shock. (See page 53.)

4. Call your physician and explain the situation to him.

Snake Bites

There are only four kinds of snakes that are poisonous to humans in the United States. They are the rattlesnake, water moccasins, copperhead and coral snake. As is the case with other accidental injuries, prevention of snakebite is the best cure. Thus, the best prevention for snakebite might be to move to the state of Maine, where there are no poisonous snakes, or Hawaii, where there are no snakes at all. However, if you do live in poisonous snake country, you should:

- **Buy a snakebite kit.**
- **Wear high, heavy boots, gloves and long pants when walking in an area where there might be snakes. Most poisonous snakebites are on the ankle and lower leg. The hand is the next most common spot.**
- **Train youngsters to keep their hands out from under rocks, hollow logs, or other places where snakes might hide.**

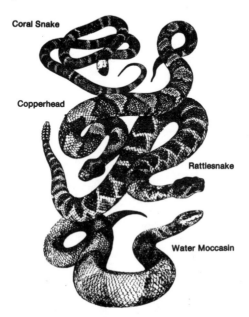

Coral Snake

Copperhead

Rattlesnake

Water Moccasin

If your child is bitten by a snake that is not poisonous, simply wash the area with soap and water, rinse well and contact you physician. He may want to keep an eye on it for infection. You can usually tell a poisonous snakebite from a nonpoisonous snakebite by several methods:

First, the area around the poisonous snakebite will immediately begin to swell and become discolored. It will cause intense pain.

Second, the poisonous snakebite looks different from the nonpoisonous. The poisonous snake will leave two fang marks in addition to semicircular rows of normal tooth marks.

If your child is bitten by a snake, remain calm. If you become frantic the child will sense this and get even more excited and upset. This will speed his heartbeat and aid the flow of the poison throughout his body.

If your child is bitten by a snake you suspect is poisonous:

1. Call the doctor, hospital or police at once.

2. Make the child lie down. Do not let him drink coffee, tea, cola, alcohol or other stimulant beverages. These will speed the spread of poison throughout the body.

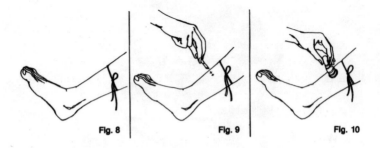

Fig. 8   Fig. 9   Fig. 10

3. Try to keep the wounded part lower than the rest of the body, thus discouraging the spread the poison.

4. If the wound is on a limb, apply a constricting band above the bite (between the bite and the rest of the body). Never tie around a finger or toe. The constricting band may be string, tape or a rubber band. It should be just right enough to dent the skin and no tighter. (Figure 8.)

5. Get the child to a hospital. Do not let the child walk, even if the bite is on his hands. Carry him. Walking will increase blood flow and speed the spread of the poison. Can you make it to a doctor or hospital within 30 minutes? If you can, see No. 8 below immediately. If you cannot get to doctor or hospital within 30 minutes:

6. Sterilize a knife or razor blade (with an open flame or antiseptic solution). Wipe the bite area with antiseptic. Make cross incisions ¼- to ½-inch long and ⅛- to ¼-inch deep at each of the two fang marks. (Do not make cuts on fingers, toes, or at large, visible blood vessels.) (Figure 9.)

7. Apply suction to your incisions to draw out as much poison as possible. You may apply suction with a special suction cup found in snakebite kits, or you may use the bulb from a basting syringe. If you have no suction cups you may use your mouth to provide the suction (if you have no cuts in your mouth). Continue the suctioning of the poison for at least 30 to 45 minutes. (Figure 10.)

8. You may apply ice-cold packs to the area of the bite on the way to the hospital. This will also help prevent the spread of the poison. (Keep ice away from direct contact with patient's skin.)

9. Watch for shock and treat it if necessary. (See pages 53 and 54.)

CHAPTER EIGHT

Cuts, Bruises, Breaks, Other Injuries

I s there a child who has never had a bruise or a skinned knee? It is doubtful, for these are the most common, and fortunately the least serious, childhood injuries.

Many youngsters get through their childhood without anything more serious than these minor injuries, but parents must be prepared for more serious problems just in case.

What Is a Bruise?

A bruise occurs after a severe twist or blow to an area of the body. The strain on the tiny blood vessels called capillaries, which lie under the skin, causes them to break or rupture. The black-and-blue sign of a bruise is actually a small amount of blood escaping into the tissues near the surface of the body. You have probably noticed that most bruises begin as red marks (from the blood), turn to black and-blue (from the blood as it clots), and then disappear.

If your child receives a bruise:

1. Rest the injured part of the body.

2. Apply cold cloths or towels to the bruised area for at least half an hour. (Do not apply ice directly to the skin.)

3. If swelling and pain persist, call your doctor.

Obviously every tiny bruise does not require such treatment. Some of them may simply be ignored. You will have to use your good judgment, based on your child's actions, to determine the proper procedure and urgency.

Cuts

When a child scrapes or skins his knee or other part of his body, gently clean the area with soap and water. Apply a sterile dressing, bandage or film-type gauze pad (which will prevent the dressing from sticking to the wound).

If a child cuts herself, and the cut is small, here is what to do:

1. Wash the cut the clean water and soap (or let cut bleed freely for few moments to clean itself).

2. Hold the cut under running water for a few moments.

3. Apply sterile dressings as described above for scrapes. (The American Medical Association does not recommend the use of antiseptics for minor cuts and scrapes.)

If the cut is larger, and spurts blood or bleeds for a long time, prompt medical attention is needed.

In the case of such severe bleeding, treat for shock. (See page 54.)

The best way to stop bleeding from a wound is to apply direct pressure. Put a clean cloth or gauze dressing directly on top of the wound and press firmly (keep dirty fingers away). Hold the cloth in place with a strong bandage made of tape, a belt, necktie or strips of cloth.

Unless there are broken bones you should elevate the bleeding part to above the level of the heart. Keep your mouth away from cuts. The human mouth may contain harmful bacteria.

Tourniquets are not recommended by physicians in most cases. Here is what American Academy of Pediatrics has to say about tourniquets:

> A tourniquet should be used to control bleeding from an amputated, mangled, or crushed arm or leg, or for any profuse bleeding that cannot be stopped otherwise. The tourniquet should be released briefly every 15 to 20 minutes.

In the case of severe bleeding:

1. Keep the wound clean.

2. Try to stop bleeding.

3. Treat for shock.

4. Contact a physician or police, or rush the patient to a hospital.

Other types of cuts that call for prompt medical attention are:

- **puncture wounds**
- **extremely dirty wounds**
- **wounds that have become reddish and swollen.**

Broken Bones

Any time an injured part of the body looks deformed it probably indicates a broken bone. If you are not sure whether a part is broken, treat it as if it were.

The important thing to remember about first aid for broken bones is that the main thing you are trying to do is prevent further damage. Never attempt to set or move a broken bone yourself. Call a doctor, hospital, or the police at once.

If the break is a compound break (when part of the bone protrudes through the skin), try to stop the bleeding, but do it gently.

In the case of any broken bone, breathing, bleeding, and shock should be controlled before giving any attention to treating the break.

If you suspect a child has broken a bone, keep him or her lying down.

If a broken leg or back is suspected, do not move the child. Treat the child for shock and seek medical help.

Sharp edges of broken bones may pierce the skin or other tissues. Therefore, splint all breaks if you must move the child. The idea of a splint or sling is to immobilize the break as well as the nearest joints to it. Therefore, use a piece of stiff material (heavy stick, pillow, or magazine, very heavy cardboard) that is long enough to immobilize the joints nearest the break. (Figure 11.)

GET HELP IMMEDIATELY!

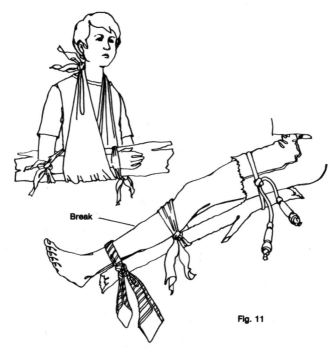

Break

Fig. 11

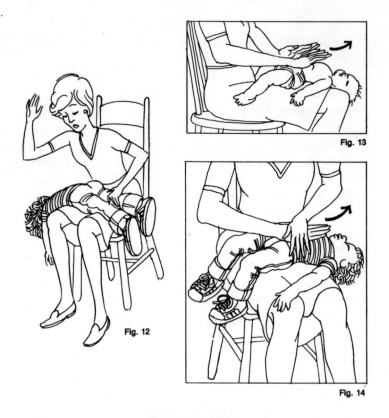

Fig. 13

Fig. 12

Fig. 14

Other Injuries

Here are some first aid steps to take in case of other injuries.

Abdominal injuries. Try to stop any bleeding. If any of the
intestines protrude, cover them with a clean (sterile
is preferable) dressing which you should keep damp.
Keep the child as quiet as possible until help arrives.

Bites and stings. See Chapter 7, page 55.

Choking. Do nothing for a moment, see if the natural
cough reflex will bring the object up. Do not try to
reach for the object with your fingers UNLESS you
can see it clearly. Otherwise, you may push it even
farther down the throat.

INFANTS. Hold the infant so he or she straddles your forearm, with head lower than trunk of body. Be sure to support head and neck. With heel of hand, forcefully strike the infant on the back between the shoulders. (Fig. 12) Now turn the infant over and rest him or her on your thigh. Quickly administer four chest thrusts. You do this by placing the palm of your hand against the lower parts of the victim's chest. Using your other hand to push, thrust into the victim's chest with a quick, upward stroke. (Fig. 13) (NOTE: SOME FIRST AID BOOKS CALL FOR USE OF ABDOMINAL THRUSTS INSTEAD OF CHEST THRUSTS FOR THIS MANEUVER. ABDOMINAL THRUSTS ARE FOR USE *ONLY* IN OLDER CHILDREN AND ADULTS. DO NOT USE ABDOMINAL THRUSTS IN INFANTS OR SMALL CHILDREN, SINCE INTERNAL ORGAN DAMAGE CAN RESULT.)

Continue alternating back strikes with chest thrusts until foreign body is dislodged or you can get the child to the hospital. Even if you manage to dislodge and remove the object, call for emergency help.

CHILDREN. Turn the child over your knees with head and face down. Strike four blows on the child's back between the shoulders. (Fig.12) Turn child over and administer four chest thrusts, as described above. (Fig. 14) (REMEMBER, DO NOT USE ABDOMINAL THRUSTS IN SMALL CHILDREN.) Even if the object is dislodged, call the doctor and tell him what has happened. A child's fragile throat tissues are easily injured.

Convulsions. Call a doctor. Have the child lie down with his head lower than his hips. Apply cold cloths to his head. **Do not give him anything to eat or drink.**

Drowning. Remove child from water. **Let water drain out of child. Begin mouth-to-mouth breathing**

and external cardiac massage if necessary. (See page 6.)

Foreign body in eye. If you can see the object, gently remove it with a moist cotton swab. If severe, seek medical help. If severe, seek medical help. Never rub or press on the eye.

Head injuries. Check bleeding, but use common sense in doing this, since there may be a fracture. Don't move the child. Ask him a few simple questions to establish the child's coherence, speech, and alertness. Watch for shock. Call a physician, police, or an ambulance, depending on severity.

Heat exhaustion. Let the child lie down and rest in a cool area. Try to keep his head lower than the rest of his body. If the child is conscious, let the child drink fluids. If the child is not sick to his stomach, administer salt water (one teaspoon of salt per quart of water) to replace salt lost by perspiration.

Heat Stroke. Keep the child cool. High temperature alone can kill or maim a child. If possible, put the child in an ice water bath, or sponge the child's body with cold water. Massage the child to increase blood flow. If the child is conscious, administer salt water as described in paragraph above.

Neck injuries. **Do not move the child.** Question the child and let the child try to move her head. Call a physician, police, or an ambulance immediately if you have any question about the child's condition. Keep the child still until help arrives.

Nosebleed. Have the child sit erect. Apply pressure to the outside of the nostril for five minutes. Optional method: Apply small amount of *Neo-Synephrine* brand ointment to a cotton-tipped swab. Insert the tip (cotton part) of swab into child's nose and hold nose shut for five minutes.

If bleeding continues, call the doctor. Frequent nosebleeds can be corrected by your physician, who may wish to use chemical cauterization to close blood vessels permanently.

Poisoning. (See page 14.)

Stomachache. Keep child quiet. If stomachache persists, call physician. No laxatives are to be given except on the doctor's order.

Suffocation. Clear the child's air passages. Apply mouth-to-mouth breathing and external cardiac massage if necessary. (See page 6.)

Unconsciousness and fainting. Caution: Any unconscious child may have a head injury. Keep child lying down. Clear breathing passages. Loosen clothing. Turn child on side to help drain secretions. Check pulse and breathing and treat with mouth-to-mouth breathing and external cardiac massage if necessary.

CHAPTER NINE

Dangerous Drugs And Overdoses

At a time when the overuse and abuse of mind-affecting drugs are becoming increasingly widespread, it seems prudent to discuss these chemicals in relation to your children.

To be sure, you as a parent are concerned about the possibility that your child may have abused drugs. How have you shown your concern to your child? How have you approached it yourself

You could be listening to second-hand information and old wives' tales and passing such misinformation along to your youngsters. Don't let such confusion take the place of reality. (For more information write: National Clearinghouse for Drug Abuse Information, P.O. Box 1701, Washington, D.C. 20013.)

Often there are telltale signs that a person is taking mind-affecting drugs. Experts warn repeatedly, however, that when adults become overly suspicious snoopers, they can do far more harm than good. One reason for this is that many of the "telltale signs" of drug abuse may be signs of other problems such as disease or fatigue. Untrained observers, as anxious parents usually are, are overly prepared to accuse their children. But if the child is really not guilty, serious problems may arise.

Usually it is difficult to tell what kind of drugs are being taken simply by observing symptoms or signs. There are some general clues, though, and these include the finding of equipment such as teaspoons, eyedroppers, hypodermic needles, paper packs, or vials. The observation of capsules or pills, or needle marks on the body, especially the arms, are other significant warning signals. All of these signals are pretty solid indications of a problem (especially since the parent will generally know what kind of physician-prescribed medication the child is taking), and should be investigated.

Behavioral or physical symptoms, however, may prove more misleading to the person observing them. Sudden changes or shifts in a person's mood, for example, may be signs of the use of mind-affecting drugs. On the other hand, they may also be purely emotional reactions to a bit of news or an exhilarating or depressing experience.

Marijuana use can cause bloodshot eyes, but so can a number of medical problems, and so can fatigue.

LSD may cause a dilation of the pupils, as well as hallucinations. Pep pills (amphetamines) can cause several side effects, including restlessness, nervousness, delusions, drying of the mouth and nose, bad breath, and constant licking of the lips.

Goofballs, or barbiturates, may make a person appear to be drunk. Large doses can also cause slurred speech, clumsiness, slowness, tiredness, and poor judgment.

Narcotics such as heroin and morphine can cause nervousness, dilated pupils and an intense craving for the drug. Narcotics are the most commonly injected abused drugs, and there are a number of problems associated with this. Infection can, and frequently does, result from the use of unsterile needles, as does hepatitis and even the plague. Malnutrition and rotting teeth are also common among narcotics abusers because they are so concerned with obtaining their drugs that they neglect common dietary and hygienic practices.

Parents must be careful to set good examples for their children. It is no wonder that some young people think they can get satisfaction from drugs when they see how their parents pop pills—pills for aches and pains, pills to pep them up, pills to calm the down, pills to help them sleep, pills to keep them awake. And don't forget that both alcohol and cigarettes are addictive drugs which people use to alter their mental state.

The solution, however, is not to lock children away from all of the possible bad influences. Although children should be continually reminded to keep away from strangers who may be drug peddlers, no parent will be totally successful in sheltering a child.

Other "for kicks" drugs that youngsters have experimented with are chemicals that are inhaled. These may range from glue to hair spray to Freon coolants. Generally, these chemicals cause a type of suffocation, which causes the user to get a dizzy, "high"sensation. Such chemicals may also cause severe liver damage because it is the liver that breaks down and removes such poisons from the body.

In case any drug or chemical is inhaled by a child, follow the first aid directions for poison gases on page 17.

In the case of an overdose of any drug taken orally, dilute the poison, induce vomiting, be prepared to treat for shock or apply mouth-to-mouth breathing. (Follow first aid for poisoning directions on pages 14 to 15.) Keep the patient calm, and get him to a doctor or hospital emergency room immediately.

In the case of any other kind of overdose (injection, for example), keep the patient calm, treat for shock, and be prepared to apply mouth-to-mouth breathing, if necessary.

In all cases, keep respiratory passages clear to avoid choking and suffocation.

Name	Street Names	How Taken	Initial Symptoms	Long-term Symptoms
HEROIN	H, horse, junk, snow, scat, joy powder	injected or sniffed	euphoria drowsiness	addiction, constipation, loss of appetite, convulsions in overdose
MORPHINE	M, dreamer, white stuff	swallowed or injected	euphoria	addiction, difficulty in breathing
COCAINE	gold dust, speed balls, coke, flake, stardust, crack	sniffed, swallowed, injected or smoked	excitedness, shaking	convulsion and depression
MARIJUANA	tea, grass, pot, reefer,	eaten, smoked or sniffed	euphoria, relaxation, alteration of judgment	unknown
BARBITUATES	goof balls, downers, peanuts, phennies, yellow jackets	eaten, injected	drowsiness, relaxation	severe withdrawal symptoms, convulsions
AMPHETAMINES	uppers, bennies, dexies, pep pills, lid proppers	eaten or injected	activeness hallucinations	delusions
LSD	acid, sugar, trips, cubes	eaten	exhilaration, rambling speech	may intensify or cause severe mental problems

CHAPTER TEN

A Guide To Buying Safe Toys

Dolls are for loving. Games are for playing. All kinds of children's toys are for learning as well as for having fun.

But some of those bright-eyed dolls, electric stoves, rattles and toy musical instruments are threats to your child's health, even though at first glance they seem harmless enough.

Complete statistical information is not available, but the United States Public Health Service estimates that some 200,000 people are injured every year as a result of accidents from toys and play equipment. Even though there are both federal and state laws regulating toy safety standards, many dangerous toys are still being sold. For your peace of mind, check carefully before buying a toy for your child. And remember that many toy- and play-related accidents are related more to unsuitable toys and lack of adult supervision than to the dangers inherent in the toys.

The Federal Bureau of Product Safety regularly issues a list of "Voluntary Corrective Action Plans and Recalls for Toys and Articles Intended for Use by Children." One recent list told of many toys with choking hazards because of small parts. Cribs and playpens with slat spacing too great, which might cause head entrapment, were also a problem. The manufacturers of a toy helicopter were offering full refunds for return because, the Product Safety publication says, "In some instances, the helicopter flew into the operator's face when it flew backwards upon takeoff, instead of flying forwards...." Frighteningly, a number of soft squeeze toys for babies were voluntarily withdrawn because they were "similar in size and shape to other squeeze toys involved in choking death."

Many toy-related injuries to children have to do with bicycles, sleds, and wagons. Children should be taught common sense rules for using these toys before they are allowed to use them on their own. Naturally, these toys should not be used where there is traffic, and should be used carefully where other children play. Roller skates are also potential hazards, and you should make it clear to your child that, before crossing a street, the child should take off the skates.

Many accidents are simply the result of carelessness, and could be avoided with a few precautions. Here are some precautions suggested by the U.S. Department of Health:

✔ Don't leave indoor toys outdoors overnight. Rain or dew could damage them and increase the chance of accidents.

✔ There should be a special place for storage of toys. This area should be where the toys cannot be easily damaged or tripped over.

✔ As soon as your child is able to walk and move about, he can usually be trained to put his toys away.

✔ Broken toys are hazardous and should be discarded. Arms of dolls or stuffed animals, for example, are often attached by sharp pieces of metal that could injure your child.

Not surprisingly, children under 10 experience more than half of all toy-related injuries. Children between 2 and 4 are the most frequently injured.

America's toy industry is changing all the time. New toys are put on the market each year and new ways of making toys are being developed. The federal government, the National Safety Council and the Toy Manufacturers of America have provided leadership in assuring safe toys for your children. But their vigilance is *not* meant to substitute for yours. You must still be careful.

Safe Toy Checklist

✔ Choose toys appropriate for the child's age and stage of development. (Many toys have recommended ages on the package.)

✔ Remember that younger brothers or sisters may have access to toys bought for older children.

✔ Check fabric labels for notices of flame resistance.

✔ Check instructions and teach the child the proper way to use any toy that might cause injury through misuse.

✔ Avoid shooting games, especially those with darts and arrows, unless they are played under adult supervision.

✔ And remember, a toy is only as safe as its user. Any toy can be dangerous if it is misused. There is no good substitute for a parent's judgment and supervision. Even after you have bought a toy it remains your responsibility to inspect it from time to time to assure that wear and tear has not caused a hazardous situation.

Here are some of the National Safety Council's recommendations for toys to use and toys to avoid for children of various age groups. Remember, however, these are general suggestions. Obviously, if your child is very advanced for his or her age, the child may occasionally use "older" toys. Do not, as a parent, allow yourself to become lazy and let children play with potentially harmful toys without supervision.

Rules, tips, and suggestions are good only to a certain point; after that, you must let your common sense take over.

Up to One Year

Avoid these hazards:

✔ Small toys that may be swallowed.

✔ Flammable toys.

✔ Toys with small removable parts (such as "squeakers" on some rubber dolls).

✔ Heavy toys.

✔ Dolls or animals with glass, button, or seed eyes (embroidered eyes are best).

✔ Toys with sharp edges.

Here are some suggested playthings:

✔ Toys that will attract child's attention. Child will want to feel, chew, hold, and drop them.

✔ Brightly colored objects hung where the infant can see them.

✔ Sturdy rattles and squishy stuffed dolls.

✔ Large colored balls.

✔ Unbreakable cups or other smooth, unbreakable objects to chew on.

One to Two Years

Avoid these hazards:

✔ Small toys or parts that may be swallowed.

✔ Flammable toys.

✔ Wooden blocks or boxes that can splinter.

✔ Rusted or sharp objects.

✔ Poisonous paint on any toys or objects within the child's reach.

Here are some suggested playthings:

✔ Large blocks with rounded corners.

✔ Nests of objects that fit together.

✔ A sandbox with sturdy, rustproof tools. (But inspect the sandbox frequently for sharp edges or objects in the sand that could cut the child.)

✔ Push and pull toys with no small parts to come loose.

✔ Peg board with large, brightly colored pegs.

✔ Small table and chair.

Two to Three Years

Avoid these hazards:

✔ Toys that will cut or scratch.

✔ Toys with pointed objects that may be dangerous to eyes.

✔ Objects with small removable parts.

✔ Toys with poisonous paint or decoration.

✔ Beads, marbles, coins.

✔ Flammable toys.

Here are some suggested playthings:

✔ Wooden animals with smooth edges. (Examine for splinters or nails.)

✔ Kiddie cars or tricycles that are sturdy and tip-proof.

✔ Finger paints made of vegetable or fruit coloring so they are not poisonous if eaten.

✔ Cars and wagons to push around.

✔ Rocking horse that is low enough so if the child falls off he or she will not be hurt.

✔ Toy telephone.

✔ Modeling clay that is not poisonous if eaten.

Three to Four Years

Avoid these hazards:

✔ Toys that are too heavy for the child.

✔ Poorly made toys that easily break or splinter.

✔ Toys with sharp or cutting edges.

✔ Flammable costumes.

✔ Electrical toys (3- and 4-year-olds are too young for these).

Here are some suggested playthings:

✔ Small carpet sweepers or brooms.

✔ Large crayons and large sheets of paper.

✔ Dolls with simple clothing that can be taken off and put on.

✔ Unbreakable toy dishes should be large enough so they can't be put in the mouth.

✔ Sturdy miniature garden tools. Teach your child to use them and put them away.

✔ Doll furniture and carriages.

✔ Wading pools with shallow water. All play in pool should be supervised. A small child can drown in only an inch or two of water.

✔ Painting set with nonpoisonous paints.

Four to Six Years

Avoid these hazards:

✔ Shooting or target toys that might endanger eyes.

✔ Tricycles, cars, or wagons which are not well balanced.

✔ Poisonous paint sets.

✔ Toys that might pinch or cut.

✔ Electrical toys.

Here are some suggested playthings:

✔ Dustless chalk and blackboard set.

✔ Simple construction sets.

✔ Paints and paint-books with nonpoisonous paints.

✔ Costumes for play and dress up. (Costumes should be made fire-retardant, see page 48.)

✔ Jump rope. Child should be taught to jump rope on a soft rubber surface, rather than hard.

✔ Cutting and pasting toys with nontoxic paint and blunt-end scissors.

✔ Outdoor swings and playground equipment. This equipment should be sturdy and firmly anchored on steady ground away from walls and fences. All playground equipment should be regularly inspected, kept free of rust, sharp edges, and worn ropes or chains.

✔ Small sports equipment.

Six to Eight Years

Avoid these hazards:

✔ Electrical toys not approved by the Underwriters Laboratories (UL).

✔ Toys too large or complicated for child's ability.

✔ Sharp tools.

✔ Worn or poorly made skates.

✔ Shooting toys which might endanger eyes.

✔ Kites with conductive string. This can cause shocks if it drops over a power line. Cotton string is best, but still can conduct electricity if wet. Teach children to fly kites away from overhead wires.

Here are some suggested playthings:

✔ Simple games and puzzles.

✔ Sewing materials.

✔ Carpenter bench with well-made tools. Use large nails and screws. Use sharp tools only under adult supervision.

✔ Sled.

✔ Roller skates should have a rubber shock absorber under the front wheel shaft for easier turning. Teach child to put away skates so they will not get wet and rust, or be tripped over.

✔ Equipment for playing store and house.

✔ Playground equipment, which should be inspected regularly.

Eight Years and Older

Avoid these hazards:

✔ Electrical toys that have not been approved by the Underwriters Laboratories.

✔ Motor scooters and dirt bikes.

Avoid these "toys" UNLESS under parental supervision:

✔ Air rifles.

✔ Bows and arrows.

✔ Chemistry sets.

✔ Dangerous tools and electrical toys.

Here are some suggested playthings:

✔ Hobby or model building sets.

✔ Carpenter bench and tools. New tools may be added as youngster is able to use them correctly.

✔ Bicycle. Teach your child the rules of the road. Make sure the bicycle fits the child properly, and is kept in good repair.

✔ Books.

✔ Sports and games.

✔ UL-approved electric trains and road-racing sets.

✔ Musical instruments.

CHAPTER ELEVEN

Things Your Babysitter Should Know

I f there's anything that can give parents the jitters, it is leaving their child with a babysitter. The first time is especially unnerving.

Is the sitter really competent? Will the sitter know what to do if baby cries? Can the sitter change a diaper properly? Does the sitter know how to give the baby a drink of water? Will the sitter treat your child with the same kind of careful affection that you do? These are just a few of the many questions that will run through the minds of new parents.

Normally, everything goes well. But things do not always go so smoothly, and it is important to get a babysitter who is competent. It is equally important that you are confident of your sitter's responsibility and good sense. If you don't have confidence in your babysitter, you might as well stay home, for when you do go out, you'll have a terrible time worrying, fretting, and checking by telephone.

The first obvious step in obtaining the best possible babysitter is to check with friends and neighbors to see whom they use. Perhaps their sitters have a free night or reliable friends to recommend. Many communities have babysitter referral agencies. When you are satisfied that you have hired a reliable and mature sitter to stay with your child, here are some things you can do to make yourself more relaxed when leaving your child with the sitter.

For the Parents

✔ Never rush away from home. Give your sitter specific

instructions about your child. What are the child's habits? What might the child try to "get away with"?

✔ Take the time to introduce your child to the sitter. If the child is to be asleep when the sitter arrives, be sure to tell the child that you are going out and that a sitter will be there.

✔ Tell the sitter about any family pets (dogs, cats, etc.) and chain them or lock them up if possible. Chances are that the sitter will have enough problems without a dog or cat causing more.

✔ Leave an instruction sheet with your sitter. The sheet should have two parts. (You may wish to use the one inside the back cover of this book.) The first part gives the standard information that will not change from time to time: your name, fire department phone, police phone, ambulance phone, doctor's phone, names and ages of your children, any special "rules of the house," and the phone number of a reliable neighbor.

The second part of the instructions should give the address and telephone number where you can be reached, the length of time you will be gone, and instructions on feeding your child and putting the child to sleep, or any special chore you ask your sitter to do.

✔ You should also be sure to tell your baby-sitter how to work the television and phonograph, and where snack foods are. This may sound like a small item, but it will go a long way toward getting your reliable babysitter to come back the next time you go out.

For the Babysitter

Here is a checklist of suggestions for your babysitter from the National Safety Council:

✔ Be sure parents leave you with notes on where they can be reached and when they will be back, and with emergency phone numbers, including that of a reliable neighbor.

✔ If part of your job will include bathing, feeding, or putting a child to bed, ask the parents for a schedule. Find out what procedures are usually followed in the family.

✔ Find out the location of the first aid kit, children's clothing, and food.

✔ Find out how to lock windows and doors and who, if anyone, should be let into the house while the parents are away. Find out what play areas the child may or may not use.

✔ Do not stay on the telephone for any length of time. A parent could become frantic trying to reach you.

✔ Do not invite a guest to visit with you unless you have received permission from the parents.

✔ Don't turn music or television up too loud. Once the child goes to bed you will want to be able to hear in case the child calls or cries.

✔ Find out how to unlock the bedroom and bathroom doors *from the outside* just in case a child locks himself or herself in.

✔ Be alert and be careful. Remember, the parents are trusting you to take care of their home and their family. This is no small matter.

Index

About the Author

David Hendin is the author of ten books, eight of them on health and medical subjects.

He has received many awards for his work, including The Medical Journalism Award of the American Medical Association, The Claude Bernard Award of the National Society for Medical Research, and the Annual Book Award of the American Medical Association.

His book, *Death as a Fact of Life*, was a selection of the Quality Paperback Book Club, and his book, *The Genetic Connection*, was a selection of The Literary Guild.

He has appeared on scores of television and radio shows, including "The Today Show" and "Good Morning America."

Hendin is currently senior vice president and editorial director of United Media, multi-media company in New York.